About the Authors

DAN ANDERSON and MAGGIE BERMAN have
been best friends forever. They live in Palm
Springs, California, and New York City.

SEX TIPS
for
STRAIGHT WOMEN
from a
GAY MAN

DAN ANDERSON *and* MAGGIE BERMAN

Illustrations by LULA

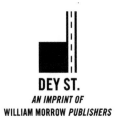

DEY ST.
AN IMPRINT OF
WILLIAM MORROW *PUBLISHERS*

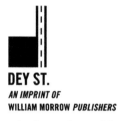

DEY ST.
AN IMPRINT OF
WILLIAM MORROW *PUBLISHERS*

A hardcover edition of this book was published in 1997 by HarperCollins Publishers.

HarperCollins books may be purchased for educational, business, or sales promotional use. For information, please e-mail the Special Markets Department a   t SPsales@harpercollins.com

First Harper paperback published 2008.

Designed by Joseph Rutt

The Library of Congress has catalogued the hardcover edition as follows:

Anderson, Dan.

    Sex tips for straight women from a gay man / Dan Anderson and Maggie Berman.—1st ed.
      p. cm.
    ISBN 978-0-06-039232-1
    1. Sex instruction for women. 2. Gay men—Sexual behavior. I. Berman, Maggie. II. Title.
    HQ46.A545 1997
    613.9'6—dc21   97-21525

ISBN 978-0-06-098909-5 (pbk.)

$PrintCode

This book is dedicated to all men and women,
because boyfriends may come and go,
but best friends are forever

Contents

Contents

Contents

Contents

Preface

You probably heard about sex long before your folks ever got around to explaining the facts of life. If you were a boy, you quickly learned that you possessed some anatomical equipment that could make you feel pretty good in addition to its use for making babies. As a girl, the pleasures of your anatomy were probably a little less obvious. But whether you shared a room with your brother or went to nudist colonies on family vacations, you knew that what boys had was really different and, somehow, sublimely intriguing. Lest you think that this is a lead-in to a classic Freudian scenario, we want to set the record straight. In the eloquent words of one wise father whose young daughter burst into the bathroom while he was showering and said, "Daddy, I want one of *those*": "Emily, if you have one of *those*," he said, pointing back, "you can always get one of *these*."

So with the myth of penis envy dispelled, the problem, if you were a girl, was that you learned how all those parts functioned from your parents or from the oh-so-carefully-worded books they gave you, or maybe from watching sequences on *Wild Kingdom*. Still, the mating hippopotami on television conveyed little information beyond the mechanics of the "doggie style" position. The female hippopotamus appeared, shall we say, as though she couldn't care less. And why not? She seemed to be functioning as a willing, passive receptacle without a care in the world, much less wondering if he was thinking, "Gee, this is really one hot hippo mama."

Without disparaging the joys of the animal kingdom, we human beings are blessed with the additional consciousness of the physiological and emotional pleasures associated with sex. Moreover, we are taught from an early age to excel at whatever we do. But again, girls are faced with a classic dilemma. Sure, they can "use what they've got to get what they want," but without full-time possession of all the tools, girls face an obvious disadvantage in having to hone their skills on temporary loan equipment. And remember, practice makes perfect.

So where does a woman go to learn more about sex? When you are younger, the only really down-and-dirty talks you could have about sex were with your girlfriends, and best girlfriends at that! Remember those pajama parties where everyone made a fist and practiced kissing their hands? How about putting on lipstick and kissing the mirror to determine what was just the right amount your lips should be parted for a kiss? How about a *kiss* kiss? And what about the once-dreaded but later sought-after French kiss? Okay, you say, that's kid stuff, what about when girls get older? We offer as Exhibit A any Thursday night in the cramped cubicle of a sorority house or women's dorm. The conversation revolves around who did or didn't "go all the way,"* what some jerky guy tried to do or maybe, just maybe, the virtues of vibrators

---

*The phrase *going all the way* was a polite way of describing sexual intercourse prior to the 1960s. Post-1960s vernacular would, undoubtedly, use the more descriptive but less metaphoric term *to get laid* or *to hook up*.

for taking the edge off all that exam-cramming. These talks are a great way to compare notes but not one girlfriend could really tell you what was going on in the guy's head, or any other part of his body, for that matter.

When you were a bit older, maybe you had a boyfriend or husband who would string together a couple of choice words like "Wow, that was great!" But such nondescript utterances offered few clues about what you actually did that was so great. Obviously, both men and women know that it is poor bedroom etiquette to point out the faults of one's partner. So how does a woman know what was great? How does she know if he liked it because of what she specifically did or because he's a satisfied and contented good sport? Ask any woman who has ever said to a guy, "Do you like it like this or do you like it like that?" and the answer most probably was, "I like whatever you do." Men are gracious and, furthermore, they know well enough not to let the screen door hit them on the way out.

So women don't have the equipment to practice what feels good on themselves. Even those fortunate enough to have had a boy toy, a lover, or a husband cannot really count on getting an honest report card or performance evaluation. Women know that they are usually not going to find out anything real from their partners if that partner happens to be a man. So what's a woman to do? The only truly accurate way to learn the sexual tricks of the trade, or what makes a guy really moan, is to go straight to the source: a man. This man needs to be someone special, who not only knows his own preferences but who has had the opportunity to know the preferences of a number of other guys. Who better than an honest-to-goodness gay man? He knows things most straight guys don't even know about themselves.

This handy little book is not written as a clinical manual, and it's not primarily designed to help a woman snare a guy. It does offer inside tips that only an expert would know. And it certainly makes no guarantees that if you learn the tips you'll be the most popular woman this side of Bangkok. Rather, *Sex Tips* is like a good coach for the sport of our choice. It gives women the inside track, direct from the source, on how to do what you already do, only better. And, along the way, it mentions some other things that make guys feel *really great*. Most important, it describes in detail how to do them. As with any exercise program, we recommend a thorough checkup with your physician before beginning. Do what's right for you, what's right for your partner, and feel free to pass on anything you choose.

If you're a youthful novice or a thrice-married veteran, you probably want to be terrific at one of life's most pleasurable activities. Whether it's with your boyfriend, your husband or the pizza delivery boy, *Sex Tips for Straight Women from a Gay Man* can only make it better. And if you're lucky enough to have it great already, think of all the fun you'll have practicing.

Acknowledgments

We owe a great deal of thanks to our many friends who have shared their stories and listened to our endless questions. So thank you to Stephen, Paul, Danny Y., Ron, Tina, Mark, Barbara and Lee, Hilary and Bruce, Rob, Carol and Emily, Loretta, Arturo, Debbie, Neil, Todd, Jonathan and Joe, Peter L., Wanda and Sandra, Tony, Jay, Philip, and *les hommes de Paris*, where many tips were picked up and perfected.

Thanks to all the folks at our favorite neighborhood bar who crossed our paths at some point, especially our savvy bartender who was wise beyond his years, those suave B-school guys and, in particular, the hot Norwegian grad student.

Thanks to our moms for being so cool.

Extra special thanks to Amy, our first student; Anna for her feminine feedback; Felicia for clueing us in on Gen-X sex; Lula for capturing the spirit of the book in clever illustrations; Spencer for wise counsel; Peter H. for providing answers to a million questions; Mary, whose Catholic school skills kept us in line; Sam for arousing inspiration; and John, who, even though he clicked his heels to California, shared many of our adventures and lived to tell about them.

And we are forever indebted to Larry and Sharon for getting the ball rolling, to Diana for picking it up, and to Kristin, Tom and Judith for scoring the jump shot. Thank you.

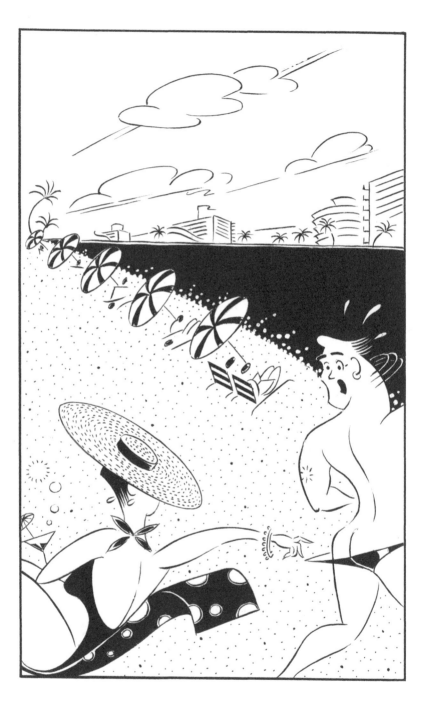

Introduction

The idea for this book arose several years ago during a series of conversations between Danny and Maggie, who have been best friends for many years. Early on in our relationship we established a pattern of close talks over vodka gimlets at our favorite neighborhood bar. We talked about work, we talked about haircuts, we talked about clothes, but usually after the third gimlet, we talked about men—how to find them and how to keep them. If one of us went out on a date, we talked about the guy and what we did, but we never really talked about sex. "Did you get lucky?" was hardly a question we needed to ask, because if one of us did, we were probably on the telephone at three in the morning telling the other about it. We were like any other two best friends except Danny was a gay man and Maggie was a straight woman.

When Maggie began dating a man who bought, but was too chicken to wear, a bright yellow Versace jacket, and had silver service for twelve and several Bruce Weber photographs on his wall, we suspected he was gay. Only then did our cocktail conversations turn to sex. It wasn't that this guy kept turning her over and poking her in the rear. It was something less definite. "What does he like?" Danny asked. "What did he do? What did you do?" Whatever it was, there was something missing, and Maggie couldn't quite put her finger on it. She was feeling insecure because if this guy really was gay, then she felt she had no chance of making him happy in bed. Why? Because somehow Maggie knew that there must be something really special about gay sex because all these guys were doing it. It's not that he wasn't trying hard, it's just that he wasn't getting hard. It was like trying to stuff a marshmallow into a keyhole. She also knew that the idea of donning a pink bustier, edible undies and strawberry massage oil wouldn't cut it. It wasn't her style. "What can I do?" she finally asked in desperation.

Although she was conducting business as usual, the standard sex scenario wasn't working. The breakthough came one day after work, after a particularly exasperating night before, when Danny finally asked, "What exactly did you do?" So Maggie got down on the floor, assumed a position, and pantomimed the act as best she could considering that she was wearing a fabulous new Armani pantsuit. Danny was quick to offer advice based on his years of dating in the gay world. While the bustier and massage oil were good for a fleeting moment or a passing giggle, Danny knew that what Maggie needed was some expert technical assistance. It was time to learn a few inside tips.

In good weather, we would meet in the park for brown-bag lunchtime lessons. We could sit for hours after work in our favorite city park discussing dates, designers and dicks.

Cocktail conversations took on a new vigor and enthusiasm. What's more, all of our other girlfriends wanted to know, too. Women of all ages, places and walks of life demanded to be let in on the action. The numerous requests for demonstrations and assistance by phone mounted quickly, and were far more than we could handle. And while

Danny was eager to share the wealth with women everywhere, it was getting out of hand. Women whom he had never even met, and friends of friends, were calling him at work and asking him to explain "the pearl necklace." They would report back on their successes. "Danny is all that and a bag of chips," said one satisfied girlfriend.

Sure enough, the aforementioned man with the yellow Versace went on to a healthy long-term relationship with a guy named Greg. Maggie went on to employ her newfound tips and became very popular. The key thing to remember is that it's not the act itself that makes an Oscar-winning performance. Sex is like good conversation: Anyone can talk, but there are some people who just have a winning way with words. It's not what you say, but how you say it. And who among us couldn't benefit from a few elocution lessons?

We remember one Super Bowl party consisting of two couples and us. The husbands went on a beer run while we stayed behind sipping margaritas with the wives. No sooner had the car started when one of the women commented that sex had changed since the kids arrived. Maggie responded by saying how vastly improved her sex life was since she took up Danny's tips. Out came a curiously anatomically correct flashlight and a simple hand job demonstration that lit up their world. Stroking to the rhythm of Peggy Lee's "Fever," we soon had four flashlights and were all practicing in sync. "Oooh, what else do you know? Tell me, Danny." "Well, did you ever try squeezing his nipples?" he asked. The wives looked at each other with a vacant, almost guilty stare. And then they turned to Danny and said, "You mean men have feeling in their nipples, too?" Case closed.

It seemed as though the women all agreed on one thing. The early sizzle, when men were so eager to show off their sexual prowess, was long past. Women are taught to let men take the lead, which is fine. But as we all know, men, and their penises, have limited attention spans and need constant entertainment. Sure, men have sporadic flashes of genius. But for the most part, sex could be reduced to kiss, touch, kiss, touch, kiss, pounce . . . "That was great for me, was it great for you?" The familiarity of lying side by side with a couple of smooches and caresses is fine, but a little variation to perk up Mr. Stiffy is always a welcome change.

Everybody knows the basics. Taking up these techniques while you're dating will surely lead to a quick proposal of marriage. Introducing these tips if you're married or in a long-term relationship will, undoubtedly, lead your partner to suspect you've been getting special coaching on the side. Tell him that you have. Tell him whatever you want. But think of this book as your personal trainer, at a fraction of the cost, and you don't even have to leave your house.

"CAN I SEE YOUR TAN LINES?"

We offer this simple line because a question as innocuous as this can get the ball rolling. When the opportunity to have sex presents itself, men don't need cryptic, convoluted messages or fancy engraved invitations. On the other hand, they don't want to be trampled like they're in a subway at rush hour. So not-so-subtle is the key. Let's face it. Most women just don't seem comfortable taking the suggestion of

Marabelle Morgan and greeting their partners at the door wrapped in plastic. Besides feeling like an idiot, you might end up looking like the last bologna sandwich left on the counter of the 7-Eleven that no one wants to buy. Too subtle, like cooking a gourmet dinner at home, will only make him feel full and much too guilty about wanting to jump your bones after you've worked so hard. The way to a man's heart might be through his stomach, but in this case you're shooting for parts a bit lower. Gay men are masters at coming up with simple lines to get guys to shed their clothes. Besides the tan-lines line, other tried and true lines you might use are:

To your banker boyfriend: "Wow, you've been working out. Make a muscle."

To your hippie English professor: "Do you really have a peace sign tattooed on your thigh?"

To your buttoned-down accountant: "Wait a second . . . let me get that thread off your pants."

To your doctor: "Would you mind taking a look at this bite for a second?"

To your new friend at the bar: "I have to go. Will you walk me home? Can you drop me off?"

To the delivery guy: "Just a minute, my handbag's in the bedroom."

To the male model you met at a film screening: Just forget it!

The variations are endless. Most men are bright enough to take the cue. All you have to do is come up with a line that works for you, and then . . .

JUST GRAB IT

We've had numerous conversations about when you've gotten the guy into striking distance but are unsure about what to do next. Sure, you can look up into his eyes with a sexy come-hither glance. You can throw your arms around his neck and deliver a deep, wet kiss. Or you can slowly and seductively massage the knots out of his neck and back. These might work, but in the end, there is only one method that is fail-safe. Take a deep breath, emit a slow, audible exhale, look into his eyes and just grab it.

You're probably saying to yourself that he'll think you're a slut. Well, for a second, maybe. But rest assured that any bad thoughts will be quickly dispelled by the novelty of your taking the lead and by your awesome performance. This *will* make him happy. A little ladylike initiative can go a long way. Just Grab It is more than a piece of advice. It's a way of life.

AUTHORS' NOTE: *When this book was first published ten years ago, who would have thought that straight guys would take fashion tips from gay guys or that a certain president would contribute to making oral sex a topic on the nightly news? But over 250,000 readers around the world have proven that, like Coke, some things are best enjoyed as "classics." So to the next generation of women, we offer these brilliant basics for handling your man.*

—DA AND MB

SEX TIPS
for
STRAIGHT
WOMEN
from a
GAY
MAN

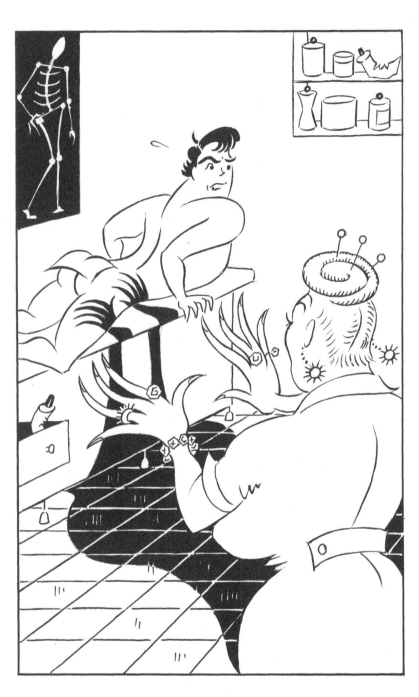

Before we get into the actual tips, there are some preliminary things you should know. Gay men look at every sexual encounter as a once-in-a-lifetime performance. While women get gold stars for having food in the fridge for the next morning, gay men know that their partners may not hang around that long. They want everything to be perfect and do their best to design the most fabulous experience ever—whether they expect to see that person again or not. So while some of these tips may seem obvious, they're worth keeping in mind.

CLEAN UP YOUR ACT

A nice shower is always a good idea whether he smells like he just got back from the gym or not. In your old life it may not have mattered, because you were the wide receiver and he was the star quarterback. But now that your hands, mouth and, yes, your nose will be in places they might not have been before—and for a longer time, at that—you'll want to be sure that he's squeaky clean. We're not saying that a natural manly scent isn't a turn-on, but no one wants to stick their face into an old gym shoe. Hot and sweaty *after* sex is good, but *before* is another matter altogether.

If you're out on a date, chances are that he took a shower before heading out. But if he just came upstairs from walking the dog or fixing your washing machine, you'll feel a whole lot better if you're not gagging from the smell of 3-in-1 oil or other unpleasant odors. Likewise for eliminating that ambient barroom smell of smoke and Scotch.

The same thing goes for you. Those silver plastic pants you saw in Vogue may look *hot,* but they might leave you smelling like the beach after a nasty storm. We're not saying you have to get crazy about this, but it does make things more pleasant.

Rumor has it that Cher, upon sighting a particularly sexy specimen, ordered, "Have him washed and brought to my tent." She can probably get away with that, but unless you're Claudia Schiffer or fabulously wealthy, do not, under any circumstances, suggest that he take a shower. This could make him feel momentarily undesirable or inferior to your royal pristineness. It is much better to say, "Hmm, looking at you like that makes me warm. I think I'll cool off in the shower." After that, look him in the eye and remove an article of clothing. He'll be mesmerized—honest. As you walk toward the bathroom, he probably won't need any coaxing to join you. If he's really dense, don't hesitate to offer a sincere invitation. If that doesn't do the trick, just say that you feel the need to take a shower. Leave the bathroom door open a bit, get naked, get under the water, and beckon him to bring you more soap, a washcloth or your body lotion from the nightstand (see chapter 2). The rest is up to you.

And while we're on the subject of you, there are a few other don'ts that women's magazine sometimes overlook.

BAUBLES AND BEADS

Did you ever notice that gay men might admire your cool jewelry but they don't wear much of it themselves?

Maybe it's true that men are dazzled by shiny, dangling earrings and fluffy hair accessories, but he really doesn't want your tennis bracelet caught in his pubic hair, and neither do you, for that matter. Even the smallest diamond studs, whether they're in your ears, nose or belly button, can do serious damage. Remember, if it can cut glass, it can cut skin. Ditto on the watch, rings and ankle bracelets.

There's no doubt that sexy lingerie is a turn-on. It becomes a royal pain when those delicate pearl beads and crystal buttons get tangled and stuck in his chest hair, or leave a dent in his skin. Keep it simple. Chances are very good that you won't be wearing it for long anyway.

DON'T GET NAILED

While men are fascinated by your fabulous French manicure, and look forward to a gentle back rub with your nails, no one wants to be fishing around in bed for a fake nail tip. If he finds a Vamp lacquered nail tip between the sheets the day after, he might freak out because he doesn't know what it is, or worse, he might think you're a total fake. Civilized gay men, and we've never known one who isn't, are fastidious about clipped and filed nails. Keep your nails trim and smooth, because you never know where they might end up.

SCENTS AND SENSIBILITY

Women's magazines are big on fragrance, but remember, they get paid big bucks to run those ads. Contrary to what the salesperson says, men do not equate a certain fragrance with fabulousness. It doesn't make any difference anyway. If they can hardly remember your birthday, why would you expect them to remember your perfume? He may like your Windsong on his mind, but not on his sheets, shirts and sofa. A well-placed dab here and there is fine. Just don't overdo it. Also on this subject, the world is now filled with pollutants and allergens to which few are totally immune. A sneezing fit when he leans forward to kiss you is a surefire way to kill the moment.

TIPS ON TEXTURE

Do wear suede, cashmere, silk and leather for their sensual feel or smell. Don't wear scratchy wools, cheap stiff lace or things that make you sweat like a pig. Another word on texture: You may never suspect it, but your pubic hair can be just as irritating on his lips and chin as his beard can be on your face. Good sexual grooming tells us that the use of a simple, over-the-counter hair conditioner can prevent a bad case of brush burn.

HAIR HINTS

Before you get overly enthusiastic about running your fingers through a guy's hair, look at the texture and style. Does it always look exactly the same? Does the feel of it seem a little odd? Don't make the same mistake Danny did. Every time he ran his fingers through this one guy's hair, the guy would push his hand away. Suddenly, in a flash of brilliance, he realized the guy had a weave. So if you're looking for splendor in the grass, make sure it's not AstroTurf.

While we're on the subject, one thing most women have no idea about is how to deal with men's body hair. While massaging or licking a hairy chest, thigh or calf, do be gentle. Unless you're lightly tickling him, concentrate on the muscle and not the surface, because an overzealous stroking may seem passionate to you, but it's a painful hair-pulling for him. Creams, lotions and massage oils can make it even worse. Use them judiciously.

A funny thing happened to two buddies of ours, Freddy and Eduardo, who hooked up one night and got a little overeager with the massage oil. Bursting from the bedroom in a fit of passion, they bounced from room to room in a series of energetic embraces, hitting just about every wall in the house. The next morning they were surprised to see their hand, back and butt prints, in oily silhouette, all over the prized antique wallpaper so preciously preserved by Freddy. Don't overdo it with the oils.

Another tip we recently picked up on the Net was the following warning: "Never tape body parts together." We concur.

CONVERSATION STOPPERS

Don't discuss things like periods, rashes, yeast infections, bikini waxing or other things that can make a straight man squeamish. Save that kind of talk for your girlfriends and gay friends. One international businessman friend of ours was dating a woman who seemed really nice, with a cosmopolitan flair. But after a couple of cocktails, she tipped her hand: She was just another bimbette from the boonies. While our friend was patient enough to hear about her Donna Karan panty hose, their relationship was over when she started discussing how her power puss punctured the puny panty panel.

BITE BITS

One last tip reminds us of a particularly disappointing encounter with a guy we call the vampire from Lancaster. He was cute and he was passionate, but he seemed to have an undue fondness for love bites—giving them, that is. Despite repeated and firm protestations in a loving voice, he persisted in biting too hard and too often. When he had an especially fierce tooth lock on Danny's back, only a swift but decisive head butt made him stop. *Do* give love bites gently, sparingly and in selected situations. *Don't* make him think that you're orally fixated, or that you didn't eat enough for dinner. And never, ever leave a hickey. That little trick grew really old after junior high school.

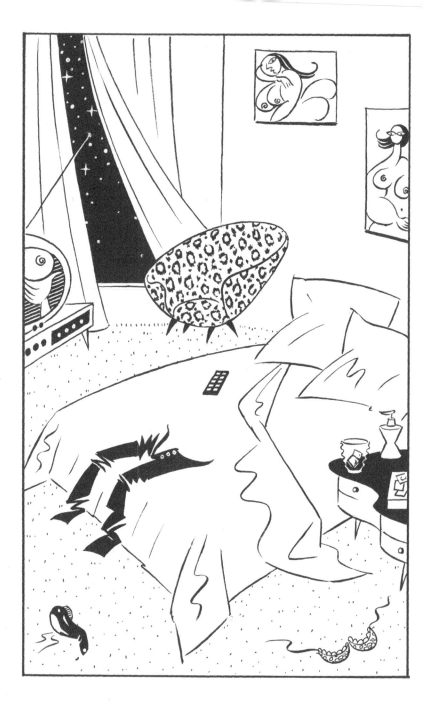

2

The Properly
Appointed
Bedroom

SETTING THE STAGE

Just like in the theater, any production will be even more spectacular when the right stage set and props are in place. Assuming that you control your own space, it's important to think about the things that will enhance and support your performance as you bask in the spotlight of center stage. One must not overlook the proper bedroom accessories, because being well prepared will make your performance seem absolutely effortless. Just think of this as setting the stage for a brilliant seduction, or having the right utensils and ingredients to prepare a great meal.

You might think that men don't care about where they're doing it as long as they're doing it, but they do care when something becomes a pain, or stands in the way of their own good time. Everyone has heard those anecdotes of passion where bed frames collapse from high-impact gymnastics, or about the guy who kept whacking his head into the wall, or worse, when strewn sheets caught fire after landing on the bedside candle. One couple we know, with a particularly zesty sex life and a fancy antique bed, used to bounce around so much that the mattress would fall through the slats almost every night. The brilliant solution was to design special steel girders that attached to the bed frame, leaving both their sex life and the design of their family heirloom intact. These stories may seem hilarious at office coffee talk the morning after, but they certainly have a way of putting a damper on an award-winning performance. Remember, these tips are meant to help you shine as the star and not as the opening comedy act.

BEST BETS ON BEDS

First and foremost is the bed. An ideal sex bed would have no headboard or footboard, so that man-size arms, legs and heads can extend or hang over the sides if need be. A few of you naughty readers might be wondering where one might attach handcuffs if there's no headboard. But surprise, this is not a big gay activity, at least not in our circles. We figure that if you're into such hardware, you're already a steady customer at Home Depot and know how to buy and install eye hooks. Besides, gay men would prefer cashmere mufflers wrapped around the foot of the bed any day. Having easy access to the bed from any angle is definitely something to keep in mind.

Our friend Eduardo, an interior designer with a penchant for beefy guys, insists that his big old bed be positioned in the middle of the room on a low platform—sort of like stepping up to a shrine. And we've heard that sex with him is nothing less than a religious experience. If you've got the room, this placement is ideal, and one doesn't have to consult a feng shui expert to find out which axis has the best sex karma. If space dictates that one side of the bed be up against the wall, make sure it's where your head is. No one wants to be side-trapped by Sheetrock because those wild, abandoned movements are physically restricted.

The question of bed height presents some interesting options. Forget the mattress on the floor except for impromptu encounters. A high bed is not only dramatic but allows for a variety of exciting positions. One person can stand on the floor with the right parts aligned to the right height for certain activities. If the guy stands, you can be on your back and wrap your legs around his waist or put your heels on his shoulders. You can also bend your legs and he can hold your feet in his hands. Or, you both stand, with you bending forward at the waist, so that the top of your body rests on the bed while he nuzzles in behind you. Another variation, with you lying on your back, is to lean your head over the edge while you lick his testicles, inner thighs, or that sensitive place between his balls and his bottom. Obviously, this works for you, too, if the positions are reversed.

Lower beds are good for other activities. Either of you can sit or kneel next to the bed while the other person positions their private parts near the edge. Legs can hang over the sides or be supported by the floor. This relatively comfortable position is excellent for performing some extended oral or oral/manual combo action on your partner. You might want to consider buying a bedside rug with a foam underpad to cushion your knees.

Any ordinary mattress will work just fine. We all know that what matters is size and location, location, location. Maggie once turned down a nifty apartment after she tested the sleeping loft. Knowing what she knew from Danny, she scurried up the ladder and tried several positions to check out the distance between the bed and the ceiling. If she couldn't sit up straight, neither could any guy who was more than five feet tall.

There are some folks who swear by water beds, so if your ultimate fantasy is rocking with the waves, have a great time. Gay guys know that the problem with water beds is that they have to sit inside a rigid frame, which can be rough and tough on skin. Worse, the frame is a real pain if it's under your jaw or if he's banging his shins against it. We do not advise it.

Ditto for thin futons, which can be torture on the knees. More important is that you make sure all the screws on your bed frame are nice and tight so you don't conduct a squeaky symphony that may lead to an eviction notice. The last word on beds is that gay men wouldn't even consider anything less than queen size.

PILLOW TALK

Bed linens are a matter of taste, as long as you don't have to waste time throwing off dozens of toss pillows and, if you must, cutesy stuffed animals. One of our gay friends told us a story from a time, long ago, when he was dating a girl. He thought he had pulled off a suave seduction when he cleared the bed by throwing her stuffed animals onto the floor. Her passion quickly turned from ardor to anger, and he was given his walking papers. To this day, he still can't believe she put her Gunds before his goods. Steer clear of scratchy bedspreads. Lose the cords to the electric blanket.

Some women inadvertently make their partners feel really weird about the inevitable wet spot. Remember, guys consider their own ejaculations as evidence of their achievement, so one shouldn't run off to bury a "trophy" under a towel. By the same token, seeing the spot left by the last guy can be a real turn-off. Gay men know that would be impolite. Good cotton sheets will allow the moisture to soak through to the mattress pad. This is a lot better than having to dry out the mattress after each encounter. And it goes without saying, clean sheets are a must!

Everyone knows that one or two strategically placed pillows can make things better and deeper. Some guys at a health spa turned us on to pillows filled with buckwheat hulls. These are great because they give firm support under your neck, tummy or bottom, but they are also pliable. Try putting them in the freezer for half an hour for a new and interesting sensation. We've found them at upscale spas such as Ten Thousand Waves in Santa Fe. In a pinch, a slightly squishier version, with the brand name of Bucky, is available at most travel stores.

PREFERRED PROPS

The next item of business is about what's next to your bed. A nightstand or small table with a drawer is ideal. Whatever it is, it has to hold an assortment of accessories that will enhance and facilitate your performance. Right on top is a pump bottle of lotion, but remember this is for hand jobs and massages only (see chapter 5). Any special lubricants, such as Aqua-lube or Wet, should be stowed discreetly in the drawer. Also in the drawer are your condoms (see chapter 8) so that they're within easy reach. If you don't have a drawer, then make sure you find some sort of small hinged container, even if it's a cigar box, with a top that flips up easily. Who wants to fumble around in the heat of passion? That's for amateurs.

Your drawer may also contain one or more toys (see chapter 11) and a clean washcloth or face towel. Women often have a box of tissues by their beds, which they might think is a perfectly fine way to sop up semen. Save the tissues for blowing your nose. Semen is sticky and, let's face it, a guy feels pretty ridiculous having tissues stuck to his penis after sex. What's more, it's nearly impossible to remove tissue bits after they dry. If you insist on the tissues, get Puffs Plus with Aloe because they're not as abrasive. Good gay etiquette, however, insists on the washcloth or face towel. A soft terry cloth is a lot nicer on sensitive skin. It won't stick, and you can toss it back into the drawer after you're done. Just remember to wash it the next day.

Before the action starts, bring along a glass of ice water and place it on the nightstand. Certainly you can sip the water periodically to wet your whistle during oral interludes, but there are other advantages as well. Having a few ice cubes within reach comes in handy for sensuous foreplay on neck, mouth and nipples. If you're feeling adventurous, there are guys who swear that a small ice cube in their bottom is a fabulous novelty when inserted just before orgasm. A word of caution: Make sure the ice has melted down to a reasonably small size, because crisp edges on the cube are definitely a no-no.

Light switches should, obviously, be accessible to accommodate different tastes and moods. The romance of candles is marvelous, with good lighting to boot. But if something catches fire it can be a real downer, so use candles in glass holders. Gay guys have a penchant for Rigaud.

Finally, unless you're planning on inviting over a bunch of guys to watch the Super Bowl, we highly recommend that your VCR and TV be visible from the bed. Not only is luring him onto the bed to watch *Friends* a good way to make it happen, but who knows what might be in store if you just happen to have a naughty little video set up in the VCR beforehand (see chapter 11)? It goes without saying that a remote control is an absolute necessity.

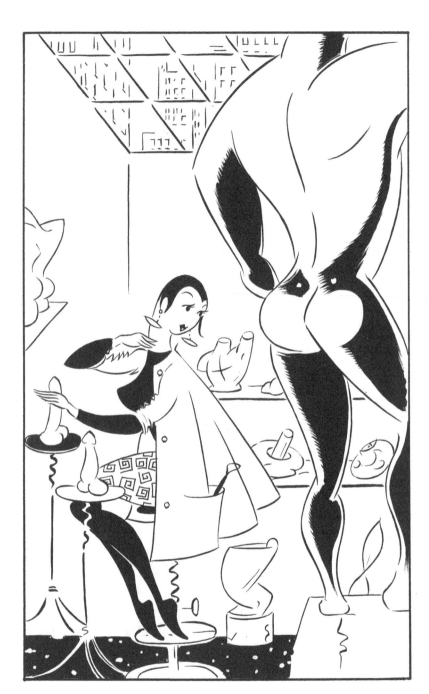

3

Penis Primer

Since you and Mr. Stiffy are going to become very close friends, we thought you'd want to know a bit about his background: where he comes from, his likes and dislikes, his thoughts, his aspirations. So here it is: everything you should know about penises, but no straight man would tell you.

"HOW'S IT HANGING?"

Straight guys may say this to a buddy when they run into each other at their local alehouse. What do they mean? Probably it's just another way of saying "How are you doing," but because men are obsessed with their penises, they'll find any excuse to slip them into the conversation under veiled pretenses. If it's hanging low, that probably means that they've gotten laid recently, and therefore, they're doing pretty well. If it's high and tight, it means they've been a little stressed and need to get boffed. Mind you, men don't actually say these things, but that's the underlying meaning of "How's it hanging?"

Just where does it hang? For one thing, not all penises actually do hang. Most men, however, can definitely tell you which side of the zipper their manshaft lives on. It's sort of like being right- or left-handed; it just seems to prefer one side naturally. Maggie thought that "it" usually went down the side of a guy's pant leg, and Danny said, "Only if you're lucky."

SIZE LIES

For your purposes, you need never ask your partner how he's hanging, but you will need to understand a little about the psychology of penises if you want your friendship with Mr. Stiffy, regardless of whom he's attached to, to last. All men, straight or gay, are concerned about the size of their rod. Straight guys may not want to admit it, but they're size queens, too. Even though studies show that men often over-estimate the size of their johnson, every guy knows exactly how long his is, usually to within the millimeter. When your partner drops a line that lets you know that he's obsessed with his penis or, rather, *how* obsessed he is, you'll have to be subtle and encouraging. Don't, for example, start laughing and say something like, "If that's seven inches, then the ceilings in here must be twenty feet high." He will never forget this; he may even plot your death. Remember that penises come in an amazing variety of sizes, shapes and styles, and that they all have something to offer you as your new friend.

Men seem to become obsessed with their penises from about birth on. We all remember a three-year-old nephew or a neighbor's kid casually watching TV and diddling with his fiddle at the same time. Although many men would probably love to recall their first erection, they were probably too young to have any recollection at all. What they do remember, however, is the first appearance of pubic hair and their first wet dream. And yes, by the way, grown men can have wet dreams, but that usually means they *really* need to get it bad. The arrival of pubic hair and wet dreams is unbelievably shocking and embarrassing.

One guy we know was so proud of one of his early erections that he stuck a little gold star on the tip, covering the opening. Unfortunately for him, the star had a remarkably strong adhesive. Convinced that he was going to explode and die from never being able to pee again, the poor lad finally had to show his dad, a physician who ended up removing the star with a surgical knife. Just the thought of someone approaching the penis with a sharp instrument is enough to set most guys trembling. Actually having had this experience must be another matter altogether. So even though you may want to give a gold star to your newfound friend, Mr. Stiffy, we don't recommend actually placing it on him. Besides, you're the one who'll be getting the gold star—or gold bracelet, necklace, you name it—for knowing so much about him!

GROWERS AND SHOW-ERS

Perhaps the most important thing for you to know is the difference between growers and show-ers. Some gay men, feeling pretty evolved about their erections, may say in conversation, "I'm a grower, not a show-er." This is their way of letting a potential partner know that that tiny little thing in their underwear actually gets a lot bigger when it's aroused. By some cruel twist of nature, some men are blessed with penises that look fairly large all the time, and only get a little bigger when erect. Some men have teeny-weeny peenies that get amazingly larger, and some poor guys have teeny-weenies that stay pretty teeny all the time.

The grower/show-er conundrum is especially sensitive for men, since they are often in situations where other men will see their equipment, beginning with high school gym class and later in bathrooms, at the gym, or at a friend's poolside cabana. To put it simply, show-ers are the men who never wear a towel around their waist in the locker room, and grow-ers are the ones who *always* wear a towel. And even though they know that their own Mr. Stiffy can get just as big as that show-er next to them in the shower, it's a source of constant anxiety.

THE BIG CUT

While most American men are circumcised these days, many men in the rest of the world are not. Contrary to what many guys will tell you, circumcision does not reduce penis size; there's just a little bit less skin to play with. In some ways, it's a moot point, because all erect penises look and work pretty much the same way. The skin on a circumcised erection will be very taut, which is why you'll want to treat it gently; rubbing it too hard will make the skin sensitive and red. With an uncircumcised guy, you'll hold the extra skin at the base while you're working your manual magic and oral action. There are a few tricks you can try with the foreskin, too, such as licking and sucking on it, which are discussed in more detail later on.

THE ABCs OF ERECTIONS

Arousal

So, you ask, what exactly does your new friend experience during sex? The first stage is arousal. You'll have no trouble believing that men seem to get aroused at just about anything. During arousal, and this may be before you even see the penis, the pulse and breathing rate will increase, and Mr. Softee will fill up and become Mr. Stiffy. The entire shaft and head usually become larger, and the head becomes especially sensitive. Our polls show men split about evenly when it comes to their most sensitive spot. For some guys, it's on the top part of the head, the part that would be facing his stomach if he were lying down. Others say that the section on the underside, just below the rim of the head, is their secret superspot.

Why men get erections at inappropriate times is another matter altogether. Sometimes, boxer shorts just hit the right—or wrong—way and the next thing a guy knows he's sitting in Starbucks with a cappuccino and a woody. Every man in the world remembers being in junior high with a hard-on, nervously eyeing the clock and knowing that class will be over in three very short minutes, with no deflation in sight. Women may never know just how often this happens to men, but it's a never-ending problem. In fact, this could be the reason why men often seem distracted in the middle of a conversation. One minute they're listening closely to your latest business strategy, and the next, all they can think about is how they can stand up without Mr. Stiffy pitching a tent right into their Caesar salad.

Way back when, when Danny was a host in a restaurant and gentlemen customers would unabashedly flirt with him to get a good table, this used to happen to him all the time. Luckily, the restaurant had huge menus that he could hold at the right angle to cover up any embarrassing bulges, and he just prayed that it would go away by the time he reached the table. "I need a menu" became a much-used euphemism around the restaurant, which was especially loved by our friend Laurie, who was fond of popping up at the host stand during the lunch rush and asking if Danny needed a menu. Somehow, she always knew when he did.

Big, Bigger, Biggest

The next stage after arousal is big, bigger, biggest. Mr. Stiffy will become his absolute stiffest and tallest, and the ridge around the head will get bigger and extra sensitive, too. This is when you'll want to be careful not to overdo it, unless you're into very brief sexual encounters. One way to tell if your guy is close to orgasm is to check out his balls. If they look tight and are close to the shaft, then that means he's pretty close. If they're way up, that means he may be at "the point of no return," and there's no turning back. The big, bigger, biggest phase can be long or short. We suggest paying attention to other parts of his body in between manual and oral action, so that you're not left watching the evening news afterward, when you were planning to watch the late, late show.

Climax

As one nears orgasm, the heart and breathing rates increase rapidly, and muscles will tense up. Like women, men climax in little contractions, about eight of them to be exact, according to a friend of ours in medical school, and around one second apart. Ejaculation can be accompanied by any variety of responses. We've seen laughers, criers, screamers, guys who whinny like a horse, and more. Some guys tremble involuntarily, some hardly make a peep. Danny says he's been known to laugh during climax, and some guys get all paranoid and stuff, asking what's so funny? Whatever your guy does, you'll want to be warm and encouraging. Hug him if he seems to want it; kisses immediately after climax can be tough, because you'll both be breathing pretty heavily. One final tip: Do *not* grab it right after climax, because Mr. Stiffy will be so crazed, wild and sensitive that he can barely be touched. We have one friend who says that he actually likes his penis to be held after climax, but he's an oddball. So don't do it, unless you want to risk having your hand slapped harder than Sister Mary Agnes used to do at Holy Name High.

We're not exactly sure why not all orgasms are the toe-tingling, body-rocking, volcanic eruptions that all men dream about. The fact is that these *do* happen, but not always. We definitely believe that it has to do with how long foreplay and other forms of stimulation are involved. The longer the action, the stronger the reaction. Keep in mind that men can toss off in about three minutes, but their toes won't be tingling. Now that you're starting to think more like a gay man, you should go for the toe tingle every time. You'll have the confidence of knowing that you were the best thing in bed he's ever had and, remember, it's the toe-tingler that gets the tennis bracelet, and we know you've got room in your jewelry box for lots of those.

NATURE'S WONDERS

How there can be so many shapes and sizes of penises is a mystery of nature. Be prepared to see some that veer off to the side like a banana, some that are thicker at the bottom than at the top, long and skinny ones, short and fat ones, ones with hair at the base of the shaft, and a staggering variety of head shapes. Head shapes are probably affected by circumcision. One guy Danny knows must have had a gay circumciser, since the head of his penis flares out with a baroque flourish at the ridge. The same thing goes for color; some get very red, but some stay the same color as when they are flaccid. If you're having sex with a white guy using a cock ring, don't be alarmed if Mr. Stiffy turns a deep crimson. Though less noticeable, perhaps, black guys using a ring change color, too—a shade that resembles Chanel's Very Vamp.

While most penises have some nice qualities to recommend them, we have to admit that some are just plain gross to look at. In this case, you're going to have to keep the lights out, close your eyes and just imagine that the thing you're about to go down on is a perfectly rendered Renaissance sculpture, and not the twisted, knotty reality that's actually in front of your face. And remember, if a guy's thing is gross, he *knows* it, so your award-winning, imaginative performance will be appreciated all the more.

PENIS NAMES

Another aspect of penis psych 101 that you should know about is the phenomenon of men actually naming their penises, but it's more common among straight guys than gay ones. Often there is a jocular tone to the name, sort of like a nickname; other times guys come up with some really dull ones. Here's a list of some we've heard:

Mr. Hooha	*Big Fella*
Mr. Happy	*Ralph*
Bunny	*Mikey*
Red	*Rodney*
Herman, the One-	*George*
Eyed German	*Juice*
Long John	and the rather
Little Pete	uninspired *Sam*
Little Elvis	(not to knock him,
Fast Freddy	though: Sam was
Mad Dog	one hot number)

Some guys we polled seem to *objectify*, rather than *personify*, their feisty little friends. Some of the names in this category include:

(continued)

Louisville Slugger

The Monster (or *El Monstro* if going for an
    international flair)

Warhead

Godzilla (which, according to its owner, is often
    shortened to "God," especially during
    orgasm)

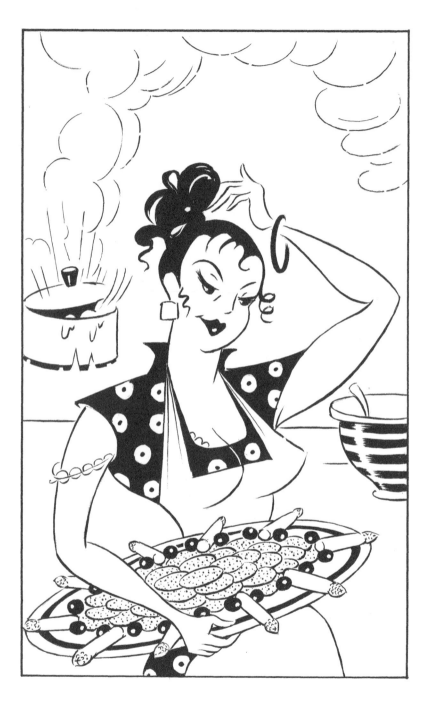

So the stage is set. You've got the guy, and you've got the goods. Now you're ready to dig into the first course of a memorable five-star meal.

Recently, a friend of ours announced he was taking a leave from his job and was moving to Spain to be with his paramour. When we asked him why, he said because the sex was like nothing he had ever experienced. This new love kept him hot, and hard, all the time. After he caught us eagerly eyeing his zipper to see if this was true, we quizzed him to find out what was so special. Was it the technique? Did they do it five times a day? Did he know something we didn't know? The secret, according to our friend, was that his knowledgeable *novio* cleverly controlled the whens, wheres and whats of their fooling around. Our friend never knew what to expect—and he loved it!

Gay guys don't think about which partner is taking the lead all that much. It just kind of happens. Take a lesson from your gay friend: If you want to win at Wimbledon, you've got to open with a great serve. Don't be afraid to start the set. If you're worried that he'll think you're an overanxious amazon, just remember that many men fantasize about being tied up by buxom Barbarellas from Deep Space Nine. Our informal poll of men, straight and gay, tells us that guys love to have their partner orchestrate; probably more often than you'd think. The notion of him lying back with someone else calling the shots—and doing most of the work—is pretty appealing. You already know the surefire signal: "Just grab it" (see Introduction). This chapter will give you some tips on how to keep the ball rolling.

LIP TIPS

There's probably not much a gay man can tell you about kissing that you don't already know. We all know good kissers and bad kissers, so what makes a great kiss? Loose lips, open mouth, and an open attitude. The fact that you're reading this book means you've got an open attitude—or are pretty darn close. But there are other places you can kiss him that will rev up his engine. He'll think you've been training for the Indy 500 and, with these tips, you're sure to scoop the checkered flag.

After a long, lovely series of kisses on the mouth, it's time to heat things up and head south. Kisses on the neck are nice, but it's your tongue that will put him into high gear. Light licks and soft breathing into his ear will send shivers down his spine. Move lower to the most sensitive spot on his neck and throat, which is along the line where his whiskers vanish. Using the flat part of your tongue, and a firm pressure, lick up and down along that line. If he's too ticklish, lighten up and move on to other parts.

Another good spot is the curve where his neck meets his shoulder. In general, almost any kind of tongue touches in this area will rock his racket. Keep heading south to his underarms. If his hands are clasped behind his neck, you've got an open invitation. If not, deftly take hold of his wrist and move his arm up above his head. The underarm area is where gay men go to town. One girlfriend of ours said that while she loved to give BJs, there was no way she was sticking her face under some guy's arm. We agree that a mouthful of Arrid Extra Dry is a lousy way to stick to your Weight

Watchers plan, which is why the presex shower is a must.

Our friend Peter is so into underarm action that he thought we should devote a whole chapter to this. And Peter's preference has propelled him into a plethora of partners' pits. There are two areas to approach. Start by licking the super smooth spot directly below the hair under his arms for a while, then go right for the center of his underarm. Use your lips and gums to massage him, moving from section to section. Another sexy spot is along the inside of his arm, in between the bicep and tricep. The skin in these three areas tends to be very soft and, often, neglected. Perhaps that's why Peter goes so gaga for pit play.

When you're bored with his armpits, keep licking and mouthing your way down to another area that's often overlooked: his inner thighs. Slide down and shift positions so that your legs are hanging over the sides of the bed and your head is between his legs. You may already have noticed that many men have a little bald spot on their inner thighs. We don't know if this is a genetic quirk or the result of too-tight jeans, but it's a great place to play around in. Use the same mouth motion you used under his arms. Start with the bald spot and work your way to the line where his torso meets his leg. Say hi to Mr. Stiffy so he won't feel left out. A soft stroke with your hand will let him know that you'll be back later to take good care of him.

A VERSATILE GUIDE TO NIPPLES

We already mentioned how some of our women friends were amazed to learn that men have feeling in their nipples.

To some guys, this is a big nothing. But to others, these petite protrusions are two major points on the playing field. Our poll shows a fifty-fifty split: Fifty percent say "don't bother" and fifty percent are nipple queens.

The only way to find out if a guy's nipples are in the hot zone is to test the waters. Lazy licking is pretty boring, but he might like the sensation of bites, tugs or tweaks. A friend of ours, who's the king of nipple queens, told us everything you always wanted to know about nipples but were afraid to ask.

The first thing you'll want to do is prime the pecs. If your gentleman du jour has been working out, he'll have heightened feeling in his pectoral muscles. Massage and knead the pecs inward to send the sensation toward the nipple. He'll also like the fact that you've noticed all his hard work at the gym. You want to get the nipple to the point where it's almost begging for attention, because when you finally touch it, it will be supersensitive. Some muscle men seem to have perpetual nipple hard-ons. Nipple King tells us if that's not the case, don't wait for his nipples to get hard before you help them along. He claims he's encountered nipples ranging in size from little nubs to nipples an inch long. Our experience has been mostly on the shorter end.

Once you've primed the pecs, use your tongue and try licking and flicking. Then softly blow some air on the nipple. The sensation of cool air on the moist nipple should wow him with waves of pleasure. Stay with this for about twenty seconds—no more. Proceed to nibbling just the nipple with your lips covering your teeth, and then take the entire pink part into your mouth and do the same. Again, another twenty seconds for this is plenty.

Now try the same routine with your teeth. A word of caution here: Start with gentle bites, not chews. If he likes this—and you should just ask him—increase the pressure. Some guys like a really strong grip, and others find that it hurts. Don't get carried away as if you were munching on macadamia nuts. Use front teeth only, and stop if he says "ouch." Another approach is to use your tongue and your teeth together. Place your two front teeth over the top of the nipple as you massage it from the underside with your tongue.

Next, try tugging on his nipples, one at a time, and then both together. By this we don't mean yanking on them like you were trying to grab the ring on a carousel, but rather giving him a series of sensual squeezes. Grasp the nipple tips with the ball of your thumb and side of your forefinger, and tug away from his body. Alternate back and forth, between your right and left hands, sort of like milking a cow. If he seems to like this, add a little tweak and twisting action to your tug, continuing to pull the nipple tips away from his body. Some guys may love this. We think it's like opening a safe, milking a cow, and pulling taffy at the same time. But if you can rub your tummy and pat your head, you should have no trouble mastering this.

A word on grips: Light as a feather does nothing here. If a guy's nipples are sensitive, he wants to feel what you're doing. Start gently, check his face to gauge his reaction, and then try a little harder. Some guys like a death grip on their nipples; for them, you might consider shopping around for nipple clamps (see chapter 11), or asking your dentist for a pair of bib clips the next time you get your teeth cleaned. Our friend, a clip connoisseur, suggests testing your grip on the skin between your thumb and forefinger. One last nipple tip: An ice cube from your handy glass of water on the nightstand can also make his tips tingle.

A FRIEND IN KNEAD IS A FRIEND INDEED

Everyone likes a good massage, whether manual or mechanical. After a hard workout at the gym, your buoyant beau will relish a sensual stroking on his neck, chest, arms, back and legs. Mix up your massages with a gentle back scratching. We already told you to be careful not to pinch and pull hair, especially if he looks like Curious George in the buff. You may not know this, but most men really like a vigorous head massage. You'd kill him if he messed up your hot new hairdo, but he probably won't care—unless he's on Rogaine. Start at the temples and work your way back above the ears, using a firm pressure with your fingertips. This works well whether he's Fabio or Captain Picard.

Assuming he's facedown, move your hands toward his neck and shoulders; use just your thumbs lightly on his neck, and then a firmer grip on that often-tense area between his neck and shoulders. Use your whole hand to knead the muscles, adding some extra pressure from your thumbs. Don't do this for too long or he may end up snoring before Mr. Stiffy goes soaring. While massaging his back, concentrate on the muscles that run along the sides of his spine and never press on the spine itself.

Keep working your way down until you encounter the

glorious globes of his gluteus maximus. An Argentine acquaintance tells us that bottom burnishing is big in Buenos Aires; it may even be more popular than soccer. Start by pressing your thumbs into the epicenter of each buttock. Using a pretty forceful pressure, rotate your thumbs while you squeeze the rest of the buttock with your fingers. Whether your grip is strong from carrying grocery bags or Bergdorf bags, don't be afraid to show your strength.

FINGER-LICKIN' GOOD

Some guys may like their toes sucked, but all guys like their fingers sucked. Good finger sucking lets him know that you're a master with your mouth, and it sends out a strong signal that there just might be plenty more mouth motion to come. It worked in *Lolita,* and it can work for you, too. The trick here is to keep it from getting boring. Start with his pinky and continue in order, one finger at a time, to his thumb. Forget about delicate licks to the tips. Put the whole finger in your mouth and suck away. Finish it off by giving him a few sloppy licks on the palm of his hand. From this maneuver, you can navigate down to his navel. Or, you can be a little more inventive by placing his own wet hand around Mr. Stiffy, while you decide what's next on the menu.

THAT TOUCH OF MINK

Everybody has their own take on textures. Victoria's Secret has made millions on marketing maribou and selling satin. We have a couple of decorator friends who can't seem to stock enough fur and leather bed throws. All their clients, it seems, love the feeling of fur tickling their tushes. We can only imagine that they must spend a fortune at the dry cleaners. We know folks who have fur mitts, latex undies and leather jock straps. So whether your guy likes sable paintbrushes bristling his backside or silk scarves stroking his scrotum, this is another opportunity for you to show your stuff.

LAST WORD ON FOREPLAY

Gay men don't wait to get to the bedroom before they spring into action. Our friend Tim, a buttoned-down banker by day, loves to pounce on his partner the second they walk through the door, before he even turns on the lights. It reminds him of his wild days, long ago, when he hooked up with a hot stud in a back room. Whether your fantasy is being a princess saved by a knight from the fire-breathing dragon, being boffed on the beach by a surfer boy, or being held captive by aliens while they have their way with you, it doesn't matter. The point is to take control, turn the heat up and don't be afraid to do something memorable.

One boyfriend of Maggie's fondly recalls the time she marched into his apartment wearing nothing but a pair of heels and her white Claude Montana faux-fur coat. It may have seemed out of character, but it turned him on so much that he still mentions it every year in his Christmas card.

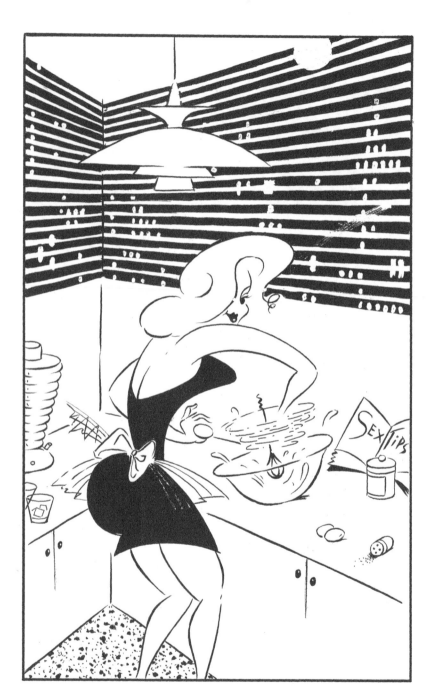

Now you're ready for action. This chapter is perhaps the most important in the book, because the lessons learned here will be useful not only for hand jobs, but can be incorporated into all aspects of your fabulous new sexual encounters. Like conjugating a verb in French class, these techniques are the building blocks of your new sexual repartee.

Several women have woefully recalled their early encounters of fumbling with a phallus. Maggie was always taught that the proper way to handle a penis was like a good handshake: not too firm and not too weak. That's poppycock. While there are surely different strokes for different folks, there are also different grips for different trips. One woman we know told us that when she gave her first hand job she never even saw the guy's penis; it stayed hidden in his pants the whole time. Even though she was captain of the swim team, she didn't know the stroke. Hooking up on the high school football field, she reached nervously into his pants, rubbed back and forth blindly, and that was that— probably about forty-five seconds, given his age. How could she have known about the whole range of motions designed to keep men at her beck and call?

THE RIGHT WAY TO GRAB IT

The big moment has finally arrived and it's time to go for it. You wrap one arm around his neck, and with the other, you gently massage his erecting penis through his clothes. What he's wearing is key, because what's inside his pants will be growing faster than Jack's beanstalk. If he has on loose gray flannels or pleated pants you'll have some room to maneuver. If he's wearing tight Levi's, be extra careful, as one hopes what's inside will be taking up all the available space. Whatever he's wearing, the movement is basically the same; don't try to grab his testicles or squeeze his penis through the clothes, because he may end up feeling like he was kicked in the nuts. Simply place your open hand, fingers together and pointing downward, on that hard section of erect manhood that's beginning to bulge, then massage it. Your hand during this motion should be more flat than cupped. Rub it slowly, with the same pressure you might use rubbing Aladdin's lamp: more than a light dusting, but you don't need to polish the brass. The genie will pop out before you can say "Shazam."

THE GREAT ESCAPE

Now it's time to let it out. Amateurs may try to yank it through his open zipper, but you're not playing grab bag. Whether it actually fits through his zipper or not is irrelevant; why risk an embarrassing trip to the emergency room? Undo his belt buckle and open any buttons, including that little button inside the waistband of dress pants, and slowly unfasten the zipper. Here, those Levi's 501s are great because you can just tear open the button fly with no risk of injury. Once it's out, he'll be so happy that he'll follow you just about anywhere.

Some women become befuddled when confronted with different types of underwear. Whether it's boxers, briefs or bikinis, lower the elastic so the penis comes out the top; don't try to pull it through the fly. Do not even attempt to fish around through those goofy, overlapping flaps found on tighty whiteys. This is a good tip if you're in say, a car, and you're feeling kind of playful. Once all those clothing layers are cleared you can probably give him a pretty good workout, although we wouldn't recommend a full climax while driving. For that matter, we wouldn't recommend this much at all, other than as a little unexpected pleasure during a road trip. Your great manual technique will be most fully appreciated in the bedroom. Gay men know not to waste their talents in a traveling road show; better to save it up for your Broadway debut.

So let's say you're in the bedroom with all your proper accessories close at hand (see chapter 2). Before you roll into bed, think about staging a stellar performance. Which is your best side, for example? But more important, are you left- or right-handed? If you're lying side by side, and you're right-handed, you will want to be to his right, and vice versa. This leaves your stroking hand free. Perfect partners would be those with different dominant hands. But unless you're ambidextrous, try to land on the side that works for you.

Chances are that unless he's what we call a "do-me queen," once you're lying in bed, you'll end up on your back. Let's assume he's a good sport and takes the lead by performing some manual labor on you. Let him go to town. When it's your turn to work on him, however, that right-side, left-side thing comes up. If you need to change sides, this is a good time to show your expertise. Just roll over on top of him, planting a big luscious kiss on his lips in the process, then come down on his other side. Now you're in the perfect position to work some magic. While this may sound more complicated than a game of Twister, it's really not that difficult. Take a more active role. Gay men roll around in bed all the time; soon it will be second nature. And straight men will like the novelty of your taking control.

SMOOTH SAILING

Unlike women, men do not have built-in lubricants. You can stroke it dry, but only with an extremely gentle touch. For foreplay, however, your saliva is probably the best lubricant, because who knows what you'll be doing next. If you're going on to intercourse with a condom, some lubricants will break down the latex. Similarly, if you're planning some oral action, the taste of your own saliva is far preferable to a mouthful of body lotion.

Although gay men think nothing of dripping a little spit on each other's parts, you will probably find this rather unladylike. Instead, work up a mouthful of saliva, and get as much of it into your hand as possible without looking gross. Start at the top and move your hand up, down and all around the penis. A sip of water from your handy glass of water on the nightstand will hydrate your mouth for the next round.

A HAND JOB IS A LOVELY THING IN ITSELF

We're always amazed to hear that many women forget about hand jobs once sex moves on to other things. One friend actually called to thank us after his wife performed some manual magic on him. He kept boasting that it made him feel like he was seventeen again, and back in high school. A good hand job is always a sensual alternative, and can be a potent pleasure when combined with other things.

However, if a hand job is the headline act, and sometimes his twitching penis will make the choice before you do, there are several top-notch lubricants known to all gay men. While a woman may feel reluctant to put lube on herself, it is essential to lubricate a guy. Your knowledge of this tip alone puts you head and shoulders above the rest. The pump bottle of lotion by the bed is an absolute necessity, since you only need one hand to get a couple of squirts each time you need some more. Who needs to deal with flip-tops, squeeze bottles and screw-off caps? Whether it's Lubriderm or a generic CVS brand, it must be unscented. Men don't want to smell like a can of air freshener. The lotion bottle is also discretion at its best, because when you're not using it for sex you can always use it on your skin. While gay men would know in an instant why the lotion was perched next to the bed, most straight guys would think you just take great care of your soft and supple skin. What do you care what he thinks?

Other water-based lubricants such as Aqua-lube, K-Y and Wet also work well. Gay men swear by Wet, noting that just one application is good for a whole hand job. We don't think it comes in a pump bottle yet, but maybe it will if enough good customers demand it.

The amount of lubricant to use will depend on whether it's a high-impact hand job or a low-impact hand job. You'll know what he wants by his response. A high-impact performance is hard and hot, using high speed, high pressure and lots of lube. A low-impact job is slow and sweet, using a lighter touch and much less lube. A final tip on lubricant is don't overdo it; if it gets too slippery, he won't feel anything at all, and your hot hand technique will be wasted.

THE STROKE

The importance of proper hand technique cannot be overemphasized. Like your favorite local restaurant, it's always there, it's always good, and you go back to it again and again. Learn this stroke and you'll have more men fighting for you than for Helen of Troy.

We have distilled the essence of the magic stroke into four simple steps: Up, Twist, Over and Down. Your first inclination will be to grasp his penis like a doorknob. Resist this. If lying side by side, the back of your stroking hand should be facing his stomach; fingers on top, thumb underneath, making a ring around the shaft. Press your *other* hand around the base of his penis; your fingers are flat on his pubic hair, your thumb goes under the base. Thumb and forefinger form an L, sort of like a hand signal to stop, but he'll want you to go, go, go. This constant, firm pressure on the base, about as much as it would take to push a heavy revolving door, directs the sensation to his penis, keeps it stiff and smooth, and has the added bonus of making his dick look bigger than a ballistic missile—at least from his point of view. Starting at the base with your stroking hand, steadily glide up to the tip. When you reach the head, swivel your hand so that your full palm goes over the top, then come straight down to the base. Barely let go, even as you

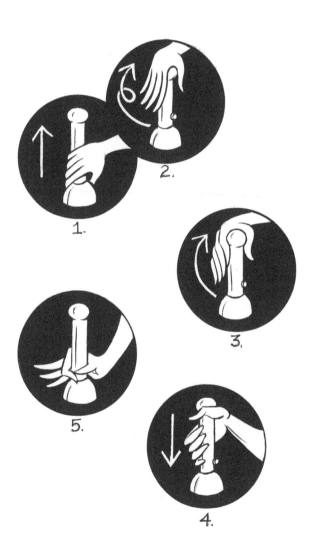

1.

2.

3.

4.

5.

prepare for the next stroke, because maintaining contact feels great for him.

One girlfriend called to report on her use of the up, twist, over and down technique just days after learning it. She said that her husband was moaning, "ooh"-ing, and cooing like a pigeon—something she's never seen before. She used her handy bottle of Lubriderm, put both hands into position and went to town. So did he, adding that he liked the fact that she was in control. We gave her high marks for being such a quick study. We also heard through the grapevine that her husband bought her a pair of diamond stud earrings that week, just for the heck of it.

So your next question is: How hard do I squeeze it? The answer is probably "Harder than you think." About as much pressure as you would use to grip a Nautilus machine, unless you're bench-pressing two hundred pounds. In other words, you want to hold a diet Coke, but you don't want to crush the can. If you feel you want to practice, try picking up a tube of slice-and-bake cookie dough. While it will be larger than most of the guys you'll encounter, the consistency is just about right for practice. Stroke the tube hard enough to leave a slight impression, but not hard enough to leave a dent. And, after practicing with your girlfriends, it's always nice to relax with some fresh-baked cookies and a cup of tea. Your husband or boyfriend will be none the wiser.

There are three basic positions for hand action: side by side, guy straddling above, and woman between his legs. The stroke is pretty much the same in each, with slight variations.

Side by Side

Gay men tend not to prefer the side-by-side position, but straight couples tend to end up this way. As discussed above, begin slowly and use the up, twist, over and down technique starting with the back of your hand facing his belly.

Man Straddling Woman

This is the position most preferred by gay men. You are on your back with your knees bent, and he straddles over your stomach on his knees. Place one hand at the base of his penis in the L formation discussed above. This time, the back of your other, stroking hand will be facing *your* belly while you engage in the up, twist over and down technique. Both of you will have a great view of his love wand, and while you're tossing him off he can do a little hand action on you, too—one hand on your breast and the other on your snatch. Of course, he'll need some degree of coordination for this, but that's a whole other book that he'll have to buy for himself. A little pelvic thrust action by both of you can liven things up even more. And you can skip your "tighter assets" class at the gym the next day, too.

Between His Legs

Another great position, which gives you maximum freedom and control, is called French polishing. This position has him on his back, legs apart, with you kneeling in between. Again, the up, twist, over and down technique is performed by the stroking hand, while the other hand presses firmly at the base in the L position. He'll be turned on by seeing his own shaft make its skyward ascension. What did Adam say to Eve when he started getting an erection? "Stand back, I don't know how big this thing's going to get." Ever wonder why men think this joke is so funny?

VARIATIONS ON A THEME

While up, twist, over and down is your basic technique, you'll want to mix in some other moves. The head rub is another excellent variation. This is done by gently rubbing just the back of the penis head, not the tippy-top and not the underside, with the palm of your hand. This part of the head is perhaps the most sensitive part of the penis; in most men the head rub produces a joyous mixture of tremors, moaning and shuddering—the closest approximation we can think of is when you rub a dog's belly and his leg starts twitching. This stroke will tend to bring your guy close to orgasm, so don't do it for too long at a time.

Another variation is to use just your thumb and index finger to make a ring around the penis. This move will feel most like intercourse to him, and you will want to use a pretty tight grip. The sensation of the rim of his rod popping through your tightly squeezed fingers is what will most excite him.

A variation on the L formation of the base hand is to hold his testicles. Place your hand, palm up, under his balls, then use your thumb and index finger to make a fairly tight ring at the top of the sac. His balls will then rest in your palm. A slight downward tug will not only make Mr. Stiffy stand up, it will also make his balls smooth so that you can stroke them. Massage them gently with your stroking hand between strokes on his penis.

If you're feeling especially adventurous, try inserting a finger into his bottom. Apply a little lubricant to your finger, massage his back door area and insert slowly. His reaction will tell you how far in to go. You can also try just massaging the area without actually going in. He may be shocked that you did this, but he may also end up begging for more.

All, or any combination, of these techniques together should make for a very satisfying orgasm. Just before he comes—you'll know this is imminent when he starts to hyperventilate and contort his face into all kinds of weird positions—move straight into the ring technique, and stroke very quickly and with a good amount of pressure. Don't move the base hand away. Allow him to thrust his hips at the same time, while being careful not to lose your grip. Soon you'll hear his ecstatic moans. Once he begins to climax, lighten up your stroke considerably, and prepare to let go. When he starts shivering, convulsing and screaming outrageous gibberish, it's time to let go.

NOTES ON THE LONG HAUL

In discussing the actual orgasm, we realized that there is an incredible gender gap in men's and women's perceptions of ejaculation. Danny kept talking about the thrill of seeing it happen, while Maggie insisted that women really don't care. An informal poll of women, gay men and straight men proved that both were right. Men, regardless of their orientation, love to see themselves ejaculate, while women, for the most part, can't understand at all why this should be so thrilling.

What most women don't know is that men compare the distance of their ejaculation to an Olympic event. Unlike the javelin thrower, however, they will probably never win a gold medal for it. But given the chance and a couple of drinks, they are apt to look back on their longest shot with the same fond nostalgia as a game-winning touchdown from their high school days. One man was so impressed by his roommate's teenage ability to consistently hit the ceiling that he still talks about it thirty years later. So don't be surprised if your partner hauls back and takes aim at those Monet haystacks in the poster above your bed. While you may not want his load all over your face, be a good sport and pretend to be somewhat interested. And try not to jump out of the way as if someone just yelled "Fire" in a crowded sample sale.

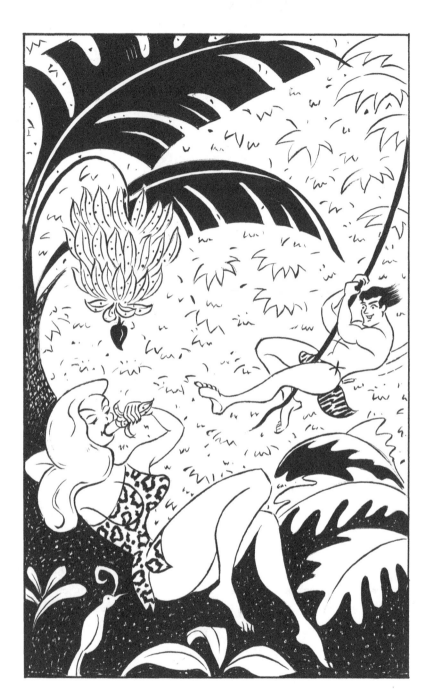

6

"You Know How to Whistle, Don't You? Just Put Your Lips Together and . . ."

So what is the one thing that most men seem willing to die for? The thing that can turn the most high-powered businessman into a sniveling idiot? The thing that reduces Ph.D. linguists to phrases such as "Oh, yeah!"? We all know the answer—a good blow job!

What is it about a blow job that makes it so prized? First of all, it feels great. Second, guys have the pleasure of watching and experiencing it at the same time. And third, they get to have an orgasm without doing a lot of work. Of course, how much work he does before or after is up to you.

One woman we know summed up her philosophy about oral sex in one blunt statement: "I ain't putting nothin' in my mouth unless I can cut it with a knife." We suggest she get a better attitude; a number of famous ladies in history have used their oral expertise to achieve great success in international politics, high finance and royal society. Madonna even showed a little of her skill on the silver screen. If you can make the most of your mouth motion, you can have just about anything, whether it's straight As in grad school or the Hope diamond.

Unbeknownst to him, a really good friend of ours, Jim, had the reputation for giving the best head in the city. He found this out one day while sitting in the chair of Jonathan, our hairstylist. Apparently, Jonathan had been at a fancy dinner party when Jim's name came up in the context of desirable men about town. Someone said, rather indiscreetly we feel, that Jim gave the best blow jobs ever. Jonathan, only knowing Jim in a wash, cut and blow-dry venue, just couldn't imagine it. It was only when two other people at the table confirmed that Jim got first prize in their BJ book also that the stylist believed it. From that day on, Jim received star treatment at the salon and never paid extra for deep-conditioning treatments.

Just the suggestion of mouth mastery will make men quiver. Frederica, another young woman we know, found a unique way to distinguish herself at parties. By demonstrating her uncanny ability to tie a cherry stem into a knot using only her tongue, she was always surrounded by hopeful suitors. Sometimes, she didn't even have to demonstrate, as the mere mention of it was enough to get guys thinking. She's very popular.

BJ BASICS

A common male misconception is that the fuller the lips, the better the blow job. We say any old lips will do. It's not the size, it's what you do with them. These BJ basics are guaranteed to blow his mind as well his horn.

The key to a good blow job exists just as much in your head as in your hands and mouth. He's allowing you to take control over the most sensitive and precious parts of his body. Deep down he knows that you could knock him off in a nanosecond. Remember, his penis is your friend, and you'll want to give it as much attention as you would your very, very best friend. You really have to show respect and concentrate big time on what you're doing. And he'll know if you're really being friends with Mr. Stiffy, or just being a phony.

We cannot overemphasize the proper state of mind. He wants to feel that you are enthusiastically devoting your talents to making his penis happy, and that you're not just doing it because you had too much to drink. BJs under those circumstances are not as memorable for him. This activity requires your full attention.

Our friend Jonathan told us about a date he went on with an older gentleman. They were making out passionately when Jonathan moved south and was about to go down on his date. Much to Jonathan's chagrin he found a mass of gray hair, froze up, and was simply unable to continue. "It was like having sex with my father or something," he told us afterward. If you think the same thing might happen to you, and you have a fear of gray hair, too, we recommend that you just turn off the light. The real point of the story is that people have all kinds of preconceived notions about and associations with BJs and that you should probably jettison them in order to fully enjoy your new sex life.

Although many people would have you believe that the key to BJs is sucking, his penis is no lollipop. The central action is to move the lips in an up and down, or back and forth, motion. What makes this act so delicious is that you can vary the pressure of your lips, take the penis out of your mouth, lick the sides and the top, and use your tongue and hands in a variety of ways that will deliver a scintillating series of sensations.

The building blocks of BJs consist of mouth only, mouth and tongue, and mouth and hands. Building with these blocks is your quickest route to a Park Avenue penthouse. Don't take the power of a blow job lightly. Know what to do, and when and how to do it. Whether it's the overture, the entr'acte or the grand finale, the BJ rightly deserves a place of honor in your sexual repertoire.

If you're starting with Mr. Softee, you should have no

trouble putting the whole thing in your mouth while you gently suck and lick. Don't start moving your mouth up and down until he's at least semierect. As with your hand job technique, making a ring around the base of the shaft will help make him hard quicker. And Mr. Softee will turn into Mr. Stiffy in no time.

Before you really get into it, take a sip from your handy glass of water. Kneel between his legs so you can show respect for his prized possession. Put both hands into the L position around the base of the shaft. Lick the whole tip, and then use your tongue to lick up and down the sides. Now it should be slick enough to slide into your mouth easily. Covering your teeth with your lips, and keeping your mouth taut, glide the head inside and lick the sensitive spot underneath with both the tip and flat part of your tongue. Amateurs may think they should use a snakelike quickie lick, but your lick should be more like what you would use on your favorite flavor of ice cream cone.

Still covering your teeth, and maintaining your pressure, proceed down the shaft as far as you can go in one fell swoop. Women usually think it's better to go up and down, letting a little more into their mouths each time. That's for amateurs. Let him know right away that you're going to take good care of him. Relax the muscles in your neck and jaw as much as possible. Try to breathe through your nose. Being in this position allows you to control how far in it goes. Pull your mouth back up the entire length of the shaft, right over the ridge of the tip. Just as in the ring technique of the hand job, he'll love the sensation of your lips popping over this ridge. Take it out of your mouth for a second, and go right back down. This will give you a chance to breathe.

Continue the full up-and-down-the-entire-shaft motion at a sensual, slow pace. Once you get bored with this, usually after two to three minutes, it's time to start using your hand. One hand will always remain at the base of the penis to keep it in place. With the other hand, make a ring with your thumb and forefinger, and follow the movement of your lips up and down. Maintain the slow pace. Remember to breathe when you get to the top. When you're ready to make him really moan, switch from the ring to the magic upstroke, twist, over and down technique, combining a hand stroke with a mouth stroke. Coordinating these motions will take some practice, but it will be well worth it. Still keep the pace slow and steady, or it may be over before you know it.

Don't forget to pay attention to his nipples, if he likes that (see chapter 4). This will give you something else to concentrate on so you don't get bored, and it will feel great for him. Let your hands work their magic on his penis for a bit, while you use your mouth on his inner thighs, balls, lower stomach and that sensitive spot where his legs meet his body. Try licking this area first to soften it up, then use your lips to lightly squeeze and massage it (see chapters 4 and 7). Once you get really good at this, you can have your mouth on his shaft while one hand tweaks his nipples and the other holds his balls.

We recommend torturing him a bit to remind him just how good you really are. You can, in fact you should, pause in the middle of a blow job any old time you feel like it. Stop what you're doing. Remove your hand and mouth, and move back up his stomach and chest to his face. Planting a couple of kisses on his lips, neck and shoulders about now will let him cool down for a few minutes. Stopping, starting, stopping and starting again will make for a bigger, better and much more powerful orgasm.

After you've stopped and started a few times, and you've got him just about ready to burst, return to the upstroke, twist, over and down–mouth combo, work in some head rub action (see chapter 5), and go into a fast ring technique–mouth combo. Gay men who at one time had sex with women say the difference is that women rarely go hard and fast enough toward the end. We're not telling you to get sloppy, just build up the crescendo to a rousing climax. When he's ready to let it rip, move your head out of the way, or prepare to swallow—more on this later. Keep stroking with your hand until it's over. Don't forget to let go after the first few spurts. It's a rare guy who likes his penis held immediately after ejaculation. Now might be an excellent time to mention an engagement ring, or suggest that trip to Paris you've been wanting.

THE UNCUT VERSION

We seem to know a lot of savvy women who get flustered with foreskin. If your partner is uncircumcised, there are a couple of other tricks that will surprise him. Put your hand around the shaft so that the foreskin still covers the head. Keeping your fingers in the same position, as if you were changing a light bulb, gently stroke the foreskin from the ridge of the head out toward the tip. If there's enough skin left at the end, you can tweak it closed, moving your fingers slightly back and forth sideways, while still keeping the whole head covered. Now you can really begin to make him moan by pulling the foreskin back in stages, bit by bit. Uncover just the tip of the head, and using a probing lick, work your tongue in and out around the head while you still hold the foreskin in place. Next, uncover the entire head, but keep the foreskin just under the ridge as you lick the head. When he's really, really hard, the foreskin should stay put once it's pulled back completely. But don't worry if it flops back sometimes; this will just be another interesting sensation for him. A word on uncut orgasms: Not only is it nice to see a straight shooter, but if you keep the foreskin down at the base, he shouldn't have to jump up and wash immediately afterward.

ADVANCED TECHNIQUES

Once you've mastered BJ basics, you'll be ready to move on to some more advanced action. Some of these positions may be a little unfamiliar to him. But remember that your movements will remain pretty much the same no matter what position you're in. The degree of control you maintain will also vary. When you're about to go into a major position change, maintain contact by massaging him, kissing him and lightly stroking his penis. This will prevent any awkward lapses in action that could detract from your Oscar-winning performance.

Side by Side

One position that is fairly comfortable for both the blower and the blowee is side by side. This doesn't necessarily mean that your bodies are opposed to each other. He lies on his side, with his erection facing you. You are also lying on your side, except that your face is level with his penis. The advantage to this position is that you can relax your head and neck because the side of your head is resting on the bed, or on your buckwheat pillow. You won't have quite as much room to maneuver your hands, but you'll still be able to incorporate the ring technique and the up, twist, over and down. He'll like this position, too, because it will allow him to thrust his hips with a little more freedom. Since he'll be thrusting, remember that your breathing is very important. If Mr. Stiffy is heading all the way in, you'll need to breathe when he's on the way out, otherwise you might gag.

69

The 69 position has a legendary status in our culture. It seems that even grown men can't say it without chuckling like Beavis and Butt-head. Even at gay bingo games, whenever the master of ceremonies calls O-69, everyone has to jump out of their seats and scream "Ooooh 69!" We all know the basics of the position. Gay porno stories are full of hot, steamy 69s where the person on the bottom watches the rippling, taut muscles of the man on top as he does push-ups over the guy's penis. But gay men know that there is an awful lot of acrobatics involved in this style of 69, and they probably don't do it as much as the porno mags would have you believe. For one thing, if the man is above you with a hard-on, it's pretty difficult to get it into your mouth at the correct angle. And if you're on top, he has to be short enough, and you have to be tall enough, to make all the parts fit together. Besides, you'll probably get pretty tired of bobbing your snatch up and down so he doesn't suffocate.

Let's suppose the heights are right and you're on top. Slide a pillow under his bottom, and have him bend his knees to bring his penis closer. Slide your buckwheat roll under his neck to support his head and bring it where you want it. You might try sitting on his chest for a bit, knees bent along his sides, while leaning forward to give him a BJ. Suggest that he massage your back and buttocks, since he'll be looking at them anyway. He'll probably be creative enough to figure out what else he can do to you with his hands. Now, you will be approaching his erect manhood from the opposite side. This angle can be good or bad, depending on his equipment, and where he likes to be licked the most. If there is a slight curve in his penis, then you might be able to allow a bit more of it to enter your mouth, which is good. You will still want to keep one hand at the base of his penis to keep it standing at attention, and you will also be able to add the ring and stroke techniques as desired. This position is generally good because it allows for deeper penetration, a high degree of control on your part and is pretty comfortable for you. Besides him needing a long and nimble tongue, the disadvantage is that he can't see the action, and we all know how much he loves to see his magic wand stand tall and proud. Forget this position if he is really tall or has a pipsqueak dick.

Upstanding Citizen

There are two positions that involve your partner standing up. The first is very basic. We've all seen movies where the guy's pants are wrapped around his ankles while he gets head from somebody. This type of oral action usually occurs before you even hit the bed, and can be very exciting in the heat of the moment. It's even better when you use one hand on his balls or nipples. We recommend doing it just long enough to keep things hot, then climb into bed, or you may not even get your bra off before he lets his load loose.

The second standing position is one you might try in the middle of long, sensual foreplay. Coaching him into position may be a bit difficult, since he probably won't have any idea where you're going with this. If he's already standing, then just keep stroking his penis while you get into position on the bed. The basic position is this: The man stands at the side of the bed, while you lay on your back across the bed, your head hanging just a bit over the side. Needless to say, this position won't work if you're still sleeping on your college futon. The bed has to be high enough for your mouth to be at the same height as his straight and narrow.

The big advantage to this is that the bend in your neck will allow for maximum entry into your mouth and even your throat. Keep in mind, however, that he will be thrusting his johnson into your mouth, and you will have far less control than you do in other positions. Try placing your hands on his thighs to regulate his movements. If he's good, he'll lean forward and massage your outstretched—i.e., firm-looking—body. He may also begin some oral action on you. But keep in mind that your head is upside down and you probably shouldn't stay that way too long, or you may end up passing out, and nothing ruins a perfect evening quicker than that.

Putting on a Good Face

Another gay movie fave is something that resembles oral intercourse. Suppose you're kissing and he's on top, just wriggle down under him until you reach his shaft. Much as he might during intercourse, he'll know to hold himself up with his arms while he inserts his penis into your mouth. He'll probably like this a lot since it comes close to intercourse, he can see the action, and there's really not a lot he can do on you while you're down there. He'll also see the rewards of doing regular push-ups at the gym. He'll probably start thrusting in and out, which means your head can stay in one place. But if he's too vigorous, or on the smaller scale of things, you need to control his movements with your hands and head. This position can be a little rough on the neck since you have to bob your head up and down to maintain a grip on his penis. Try slipping your buckwheat pillow under your neck and it should be smooth sailing from there.

ADD-ONS

There are a few little extras worth mentioning here that will ensure that your performance goes from Oscar-nominated to award winner. They can be incorporated into the BJ at any point, and the added variation will be fun for you to try and great for him to feel.

Dick Whipping

Don't worry; we're not talking leather crops here. Perhaps a better term might be dick slapping, although that sounds pretty intimidating, too. The movement is simply this: As you slide his shaft out of your mouth, flick his penis against your cheek or neck for a couple of gentle, and we mean gentle, slaps. Try it a little bit harder if he seems to enjoy it. The point of this is not that it's "rough sex" or anything, it's simply another sensation that will feel good and round out your best BJ technique. It also gives you a chance to breathe and recoup for your next round of oral action.

Hummers

A hummer is another light sensation that he will enjoy. A hummer is really just a moan or hum during the BJ, which will create a slight vibration in your throat and, in turn, on his penis. We're not saying that you need to belt out four bars of "Don't Cry for Me, Argentina" during sex, just a low hum or moan in your throat will do nicely. Try changing the pitch of your hum to vary the sensation.

Tinglers

A tingler requires a little advance work, because you'll need a supply of cinnamon or minty mouthwash nearby. Put a small amount in your mouth; remember that you don't want to end up swallowing it. As you go back down on him, release the mouthwash slowly so that it drips down his shaft. The tingly sensation will drive him wild, and it has the added bonus of preventing "dick breath" (see below) when you move back to kiss him on the lips.

Your handy glass of water with ice will add yet another

super sensation. During one of your delicate sips amidst the oral action, take an ice cube in your mouth. When you go back down on him, the combination of cold ice and the warmth of your mouth will drive him into ecstasy. As the ice melts, it will also keep him well-lubed for extended oral activity. If you're feeling really adventurous, try taking the cube out of your mouth and sliding it up and down his manshaft. The warmth of your mouth after that will feel like a cashmere blanket to him, so this might also be a good time to mention how much you'd like a Chanel cashmere twin set.

LAST WORD

Perhaps your biggest concern about the world's best BJ is gagging. Well, there are times when smaller can be infinitely more manageable. There is no surefire way we know of to completely prevent gagging every time. A lot of it has to do with your relaxation level, and how comfortable you feel. A lot has to do with the control of your breathing. The tips in this book are designed to make you feel confident and in control no matter what you are doing, or with whom you are doing it. Relax your muscles. Your first reaction when a hot rod is heading toward the back of your throat is to tense up. Remember that Mr. Stiffy is your friend and that he will only feel as comfortable as you do. Also, the less your neck and head are bent, the more room you will have to fit his penis inside your mouth. The best way to prevent gagging is to coordinate your breathing with the in-and-out movements. Take a deep breath in while you can, then release it through your nose as you go back down on your partner.

A NOTE ON SWALLOWING

Gay men never swallow. Yes, you heard it here, and it may not be true 100 percent of the time, but for the most part, they don't. Besides being somewhat unsafe, it also takes away the thrill of seeing someone ejaculate. We know that to some of you, that thrill is on a par with seeing a *National Geographic* special on penguins, and Maggie insists that she gets absolutely nothing out of seeing a man come. Swallowing for women is a thorny issue. Some straight men make a big deal out of it, but that seems inconsequential to us. Without getting into a whole big discussion on the power politics of swallowing, we're here to tell you that you should *never* do anything you don't want to. If you choose to swallow, that is your decision. If you choose not to, then you certainly have nothing to apologize for. Especially since you will have just given him the most spectacular, mind-blowing, spine-tingling BJ he's ever had.

AFTERWORD

Gay men generally don't worry about this, but some women we know are concerned about "dick breath" when they kiss their partner after going down on him. This is another of those preconceptions that you should really let go of. Assuming you're both tidy and have showered within a reasonable amount of time, you shouldn't have too much to worry about. If you're absolutely nuts about it, try taking a sip of water or wine before kissing him. And if he thinks it's gross, just remember that it was his dick, after all.

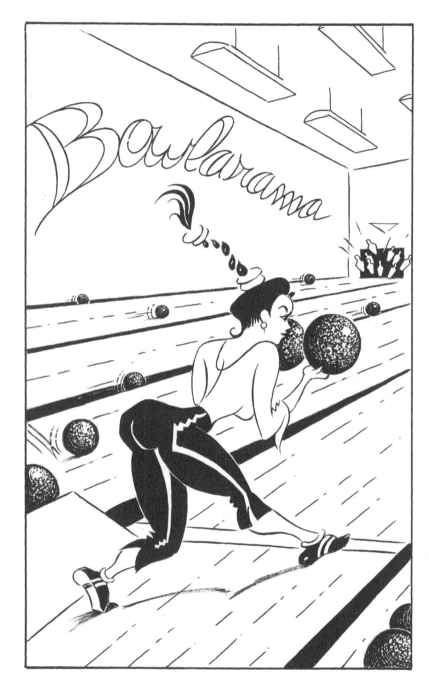

Now that you've passed penis preliminaries, you should feel pretty confident that your sexpertise will blow away the competition. By all means, keep practicing. Undoubtedly, your partner's heavy breathing and occasional gasps will let you know what he likes best. He may even start to tell you; but remember that men, straight or gay, don't always communicate with words. Stay alert, and don't get sloppy.

This chapter will introduce you to something that most men feel women know nothing about. All that's about to change. Why women are mystified by testicles is something men just can't comprehend. Danny thinks it's because so much has been made of men's fear of a kick in the nuts. But this doesn't mean you should ignore them; just use your newly acquired tips and handle the fragile merchandise gently. Granted, you may think they're crinkly and weird, but that sorry-looking sac of sex stuff under your straight and narrow friend can be a potent player in your partner's pleasure. One man we know loves his balls so much that he can have an orgasm without even touching his penis. Regardless of what you might think, the image of his balls slapping back and forth against your backside or chin is a very exotic and sensual thought to a guy.

We believe that balls have always been treated like unwelcome country cousins. You recognize them when they show up at the door, but you're not so happy to see them because you have absolutely no idea of what would keep them entertained. Women tend to overlook testicles entirely. Maybe this is because the only time they hear men refer to their balls is when they refer to someone as a ball buster, or when they've contracted a bad case of jock itch. But most men realize the importance of ball play and, in the locker room, when they're not snapping each other with wet towels, they usually refer to sex as balling. Even though everyone from Sigmund Freud to *Playgirl* would have you believe that sex is all about dick, listen to your gay friends. They have balls, and they know what to do with them. So turn those country cousins into guests of honor. We'll teach you to play ball like a major leaguer.

BASIC BALLDOM

First, you need to understand this unique equipment before you step up to the batter's box. We all know that there are few things a man fears more than a punch in the balls. Because this fear is so ingrained, your partner may even be a little nervous when you begin to grasp him there. Your gentle touch will reassure him that you have no intention of snipping them off. Once you've established the proper grip, he may like you to handle his balls a little more roughly.

There is no other place on the body that must be treated with such delicacy. The extreme sensitivity and vulnerability of the testicles is probably why play ball techniques can be so satisfying. You really have to know what you're doing here, since pleasure can turn to pain with a flick of the wrist. When in doubt, err on the side of caution and handle with care. Although there are two testicles, you must think of the sac as one unit. Never squeeze them so that they separate. This could hurt big time.

TROPHY WINNERS

Just like the variety of balls gleaming on the racks of your local bowling alley, testicles come in different sizes, weights and finishes. They can be smooth, fuzzy or hairy, and vary in size and shape from man to man. They're even subject to the effects of gravity as a guy gets older. As any league bowler will tell you, good form is just the first step toward winning a trophy. The topspin from these tips will rock his pins every time.

Straight and gay guys usually don't dwell too much on the size of their own balls like they do, say, on the size of their magic wands. But ball size is a positive guy-talk metaphor for masculine traits like guts and courage. "Do you believe he had the *balls* to ask his boss for a raise after last year's lousy P and L statements?" is a form of respect, and one that definitely affirms the notion of bigger being better. Gay men are a bit more up-front about this and use terms such as basket or box to describe the whole package. The notion is that a big box equals a big penis, but this is not necessarily the case.

A few quick words about hair: Granted, we're well aware that men in certain gay circles try to emulate the stars in porn flicks, who invariably have smooth, hairless balls. Some say that hair-free balls look bigger and are more sensitive to the touch. We just figure that porn movie moguls want to capture every nuance of action to satisfy their audience, and that it's probably tough for a camera person to focus in on a dark area. So movie balls are shaved, and probably covered with makeup, for that matter. There are, however, those who shave their balls, and we even know one poor guy who was red and raw for a week after using an over-the-counter depilatory. We still affectionately refer to him as the Hostess Sno-Ball. Nonetheless, most straight guys will not have engaged in these activities, so you will confront a modicum of hair. Our advice to you is simple. Get over it! You have hair and so does he.

ALTERED STATES

Women need to know that balls change shape, size, consistency and even location at different times. This may sound odd, but there's really nothing in the female anatomy to compare this to, so you'll have to believe us. Sometimes, such as when they're warm, for example, balls hang low and loose. Other times, when they're cold, or about to explode, they're high and tight. At the beginning of your sexual encounter, his balls are likely to be loose, making them easy for you to hold and fondle.

Regardless of hairiness, balls have a baby-smooth spot on the underside. Just stroking him softly there will make him moan. If you're sitting side by side, gently slide your hand beneath his balls, and use your middle finger to reach this spot with a light tickle touch. Use the other hand to stroke his penis. While we don't recommend this for driving in a car, it's a great way to let him know that you're feeling frisky while you're watching TV together. Just remember to be careful of your nails, or ecstasy will turn to agony pretty quickly.

PLAY BALL TECHNIQUES

The first and most important tip is that you should hold the balls in a way that will keep them from being unwieldy. We've already told you a preferred way to hold them (see chapter 5) by making a ring around the top of the sac with your thumb and forefinger. Again, perfect your grip with inanimate objects before tackling the real thing. Since we had no friends willing to offer themselves as guinea pigs, Maggie created a reasonable facsimile for hands-on practice by dropping two small, peeled hard-boiled eggs into a small plastic bag. The objective of this grip is to keep the balls together in one neat unit, but this technique also has the added advantage of smoothing out the crinkly skin.

Once you perfect the basic ring-around-the-sac hold, you can use this technique to supplement your fabulous new manual skills. Just as some women like a hand on their breast while the guy's other hand, or mouth, is down south, some guys will love having their penis and balls get equal attention. This will probably be a new delight for couples who have been together for some time, and a definite plus for new partners. Besides, he'll be so surprised that you even thought about his balls, you will forever hold a revered place of honor in the mythic rating book that all guys keep in the back of their minds.

If the man is on his back, with the woman kneeling between his legs or straddling his thighs, it's possible to use one's dominant hand for tossing him off while the other hand circles the sac and cups the balls from beneath. This also works if the woman is on her back with the guy straddling her waist. One hand pumps while the other hand fondles. Granted, this will take a bit of coordination, but you *can* do it with practice. Just make sure you close your eyes if you're directly in the line of fire. The same sac-holding technique works perfectly as an accompaniment to oral activities.

Now for some advanced tips that will send him into ecstasy. You can vary your foreplay and spice up a massage by having him lie on his back as you lick, kiss and tickle him all over. Undoubtedly, Mr. Stiffy will begin his skyward ascension. Very softly, and with the fleshy part of your fingers, start at the top of his penis and glide your fingers all the way down the underside, continuing onto the top of his balls, just like you would stroke a cat. His dick may be twitching so much that you might have to hold it down with one hand as you work your up-and-down magic with the other. Continue this delicious teasing, going back and forth, until he can't stand it, or until you're both so hot that it's time to move on to the grand finale.

Another place you may not know about is what gay guys call the "taint," as in "t'ain't your balls, t'ain't your bottom." This little spot located between his testicles and back door is exquisitely sensitive. Stroking, lightly scratching, or even massaging him here can send him over the edge faster than you can say Niagara Falls. So you may want to save this maneuver until you're ready to open the floodgate.

CONSTANT COMMENT

Returning to our informal poll of straight men, lots of them said that a woman had licked their balls, but not one man could remember any woman putting both of his balls into her mouth at once. Until our friend Laurie tried it, she just couldn't fathom all that stuff in her mouth at once. But with the ring-around-the-sac technique holding the balls together, and with a little practice, she agreed this was totally doable. In gay circles, this common practice is often referred to as teabagging. This can easily be adapted into your repertoire by having the man straddle above with his testicles dangling over your mouth. Use one hand to circle the top of the sac and gently pull down to bring the balls together into that neat package. Being extremely careful to cover your teeth with your lips, take his sac into your mouth and give him a licking he'll never forget. We guarantee he'll think you are the coolest and most creative lover he's ever had, and he'll probably be much more adventurous when it's his turn to please you.

By this time, we hope we've convinced you of the importance of paying attention to his *cojones*. There is no doubt about it, men like having their balls held, licked and stroked. But there's one last tip we'd like to mention. Play ball techniques should not be limited to foreplay, manual and oral activities. Holding a guy's balls during intercourse may require a bit of coordination, but you don't really need to be an Olympic athlete, or have arms as long as an ape. If he's on top, reach down either under your leg or between the two of you and gently grab them. The further up a woman's legs are pulled, the easier it is to gain access. If you're on top, try to control any jerky movements. Your hand grip should be firm enough to let him know you're there, but not so tight as to restrict the thrusting motions. And by all means, let go when things get really acrobatic, or as soon as he begins to climax. You've already scored as the most valuable player in this ball game.

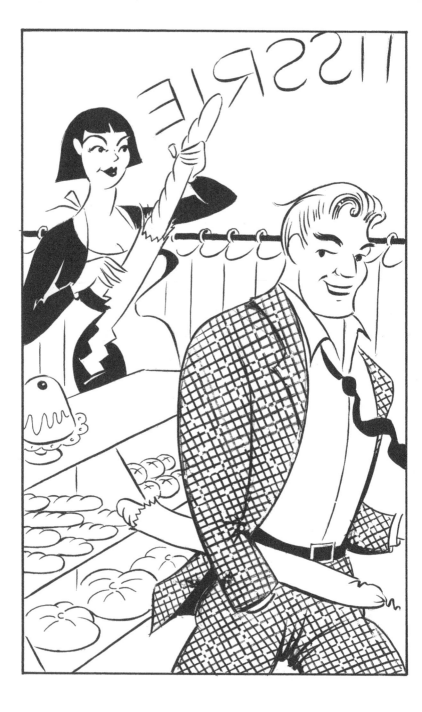

WHY

Unless you've been under a rock for the last ten years, you know that condoms are now *de rigeur* and have had quite a resurgence in popularity. Not including water-filled window launchings, a favorite pastime of prepubescent and fraternity boys, condoms serve two purposes. They keep you from getting sick and they keep you from getting pregnant. If your situation is such that you needn't think about such things, you are fortunate, indeed. If you plan to stick to some of the interesting safe sex alternatives we offer, no problem. But for those who will be confronting the reality of rubber, we offer these tips. Even if a guy is totally responsible, dealing with condoms poses several possible situations you may have to handle and overcome. Gay men are eminently qualified to offer tips you can really use.

WHO

Every situation is different, and you know best about which guys in your bed do or don't require this equipment. Some straight men wonder if they'll be perceived as overly cocky if they just happen to have a condom around. Gay men don't give this a second thought and neither should you. The rule of thumb is that if you're at his place, he should have condoms handy, and vice versa when you're on your own turf. Consider it being a well-prepared host or hostess. But since we all know that straight guys can be lousy hosts, you have to be ready for action wherever you may be.

If the situation arises at your place and you don't hear the rustle of foil, just reach for your bedside condom container (see chapter 2). A word of advice here: Even if you purchased a case of condoms in preparation for entertaining the new first-year law class, it's probably wise to keep only a reasonable number, say two to four, in the container by your bed. Gay men realize that their partners have sex with others. Straight men, on the other hand, don't want to think that you're entertaining the troops, so it's best to appear prepared but not professional. As a matter of fact, it's a good idea to separate each condom from the perforated strip beforehand, like stamps, so your partner doesn't feel like he's taking a number at the bakery on a Sunday morning.

If you end up at his place, a little advance work is necessary. On a first-time visit, he will probably show you around. This is a good time to scope things out. You can hang up your coat, but hold on to your handbag. Almost immediately he'll turn on the stereo and ask if you want a beverage. This would be a good time to ask for your glass of ice water. You can pretty much bet that the action will take place wherever two people can be horizontal and still hear the music. Plop down your handbag somewhere around this area. In the event that he grabs you as soon as he gets to the bedroom part of the tour, your handbag is still with you, and you can fling it somewhere near the bed in a fit of passion. It doesn't matter if this is your first visit or not. If he doesn't make the move to get a condom, just do it! You'll know when the moment is right.

WHEN

It may be that wearing a condom doesn't feel as great as skin to skin, but in this day and age, riding bareback is definitely not an alternative. Suppose you encounter a guy who whines because he doesn't want to wear one. You may find it hard to believe that some guys think they're being totally original when they say, "It's like taking a shower with a raincoat on." Besides being really stupid, this negative analogy equates a condom with an article of clothing one wears in nasty weather. You must redirect this fashion thinking immediately, and concentrate on other articles of clothing that bring to mind positive, fun and pleasurable associations. The best argument we've heard goes something along these lines: "You wouldn't go running without your sneakers, skating without skates or diving without a wet suit, would you?" You need to wear the right gear for the activity. And that's exactly what this is about—getting all dressed up appropriately to go to the party. Even your macho, hot-to-trot Latin lover will understand that he has to wear a party sombrero if he wants to go to the fiesta.

WHAT

While any port will do in a storm, an informal poll says the condom of choice is a brand called Kimono. The Micro Thin Plus type is especially nice for him. Kimono condoms come in all sorts of varieties to suit any preference. Lifestyles brand is also recommended. And, for your purposes, these are a little more ladylike than Trojans, Ramses or some other butch-sounding brand names.

Kimono also makes a product called Aqua-Lube, which is perfect for inside and out except that it doesn't come in a pump bottle yet. Never use Vaseline, because it can break down the latex in the condom. Never use products with fragrance, because they can be irritating to both of you. Avoid condoms with extra spermicide, such as nonoxynol 9, if either of you begins to burn or itch. Lambskin condoms are old hat and don't protect against disease. We don't recommend them. But . . . one guy we know was truly creative when his receptive partner said that he had an allergy to latex. Our friend sprang into action and put a lambskin condom over a latex one. This, in gay circles, is known as a "double bagger," but you have to be careful that they don't rub together and break, or that they're not so lubed up that they can slide right off.

A while back, there was a big marketing push for condoms with bumps and ridges. One ad in men's magazines used to promise "a thousand tiny fingers urging a woman to let go." If speed bumps make you tingle, then go ahead, knock yourself out. But he couldn't care less.

Ditto on the "artistic" varieties, unless these fall in line with a particularly festive theme for the evening. Of course, there are always some guys who like to feel like GI Joe when they wear camouflage condoms that boast "don't let them see you coming." Maybe you've known a couple of bozos who like the carnival colors? Or the scout troop leader who went wild for the glow-in-the-dark kind? These are novelties and should be treated as such. More important, these things are often of inferior quality. Unless you're partying with Homer Simpson, forget the costumes and cutesy stuff.

If you are in a tryst where your partner presents you with a flavored condom, that's your cue for some super-safe oral action. Remember, he's not the one who's going to be tasting it. If you're going to make this part of your regular repertoire, try a brand called Kiss of Mint, which doubles as a light breath freshener.

WHERE

If you are traveling, and that could mean being on a date across town, keep a couple of condoms handy and accessible in the same way that you would a wallet, passport or camera. You never know when a great photo opportunity will arise. Maybe you'll end up at his place after a date. If he never has anything but beer in the fridge, don't expect him to have condoms either. It's a lot more convenient to make one magically appear from your handbag than have him frantically search a backpack from his last camping trip.

HOW

Some straight guys have fantasies about their partner applying a condom with her mouth. Gay guys don't mess around with this much. If you must, practice on an inanimate object before you tackle the real thing. And remember, use your lips and not your teeth.

Once that is out of the way, the next insider's tip is crucial because this little bit of knowledge will separate you from the rest of the pack. Although we recommend prelubricated condoms for intercourse, you may also want to put a little dab of your water-based lubricant *inside* the top of the condom right before you unroll it because it will make the experience more pleasurable for him. Use just a drop; the idea is to get a small glob on the head of his penis without rubbing it all around the shaft, because you don't want the condom to slip off. You'll never have a problem getting it on him again, and he'll wonder why he didn't think of it before.

So what's the proper application etiquette? Opening the package, but not removing the condom, before you actually start fooling around will help things run smoothly when it's time to stick it in. Don't do it more than a few minutes in advance or the condom will dry out. If he wants to put it on himself, just let him. If you want to make him feel that his erection is the most magnificent thing you've ever seen, kneel down between his legs while you adopt an attitude of solemn worship—sort of like saluting the flag. Since condoms are rolled up, it will take a little practice to figure out which side is the top. Put a dab of lubricant inside the unrolled condom or on the head of his twitching member. Place the condom on the penis head and pinch the rubber tip between your thumb and forefinger to allow some space for what's to come. Then unfurl the rest, climb on board and go to town. He will have wonderful thoughts of you rallying 'round his mast.

You shouldn't even have to think about disposal, because he should know well enough to flush the evidence down the toilet. If he leaves it lying on your floor, or stuck to your wastebasket, think about dumping him. Our not-so-scientific studies would indicate that he's a pig.

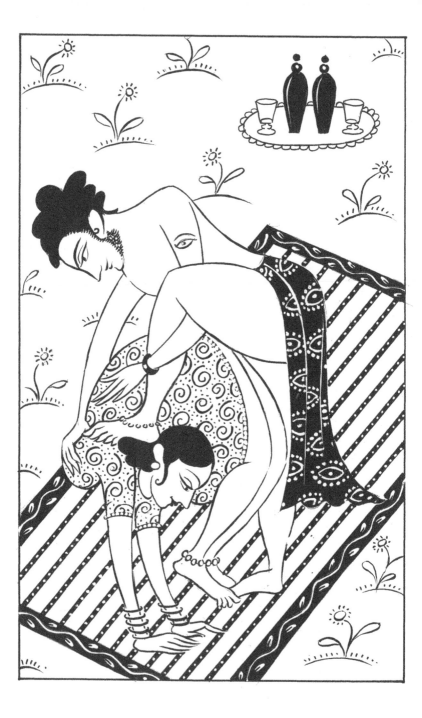

9

Interchange on Intercourse

After all of the aforementioned, his perky penis will be perfectly piqued for penetration.

Danny was amazed that most of his women friends think of the penis as one solid hunk o' burning love. They never really thought about all the penis possibilities, and couldn't possibly know how different positions feel to a guy. This goes back to fully appreciating the versatile virtues of your dear friend, Mr. Stiffy. Some women think that any old up-and-down pumping motion will do, so they let the guy choose the angle and stroke. Gay men know that every move jostles his joystick differently. That's why they vary things a lot, and aren't shy about switching things around midstream. Remember, it's not just about getting off; it's like the difference between frozen fish sticks and fresh Dover sole.

TRACK AND FIELD

As every runner knows, there's a different strategy for winning sprints, relays and marathons. If you're running the Boston marathon, you don't blast off in the beginning, or you'll have no fuel left for the finish. Likewise, a sprinter knows that he's got to fly out fast and furious if he wants to grab the gold. Whatever your mark, these tips will get you ready, set and going all the way.

Sprints

Although everyone likes to sit down to a full meal, there are times that eating on the run satisfies you just as well and more quickly. Everybody loves a quickie once in a while. For gay men, a quickie usually means a hot and hasty hand job. For straight folks, a quickie can be anything from a morning eye-opener to a midday snack, whether it's during a wake-up whiz-bang, a frequent flight or a little elevator ecstasy. If Mr. Stiffy pops up eager as a beaver before you've opened your eyes, by all means, get him in, get him off, and get him on his way. Your beau will be beaming, and you'll still have plenty of time to fix your face and handle your hair. Remember, men are always ready for sex and it's a great way, says Maggie, for you to start your day, too.

Relays

Each leg of a relay race propels you to the finish line. Gay guys know that each segment of a sexual encounter has equal importance. In a relay race, each runner holds the baton for a certain segment, but in this case you're the only contestant, so *you* have to set the pace or his baton may drop before you reach the finish line. If you're combining techniques, and by this time you'll be a pro, you'll want to give his rod a rest in between, or it'll be no match for your snatch. So how long do you wait, and what do you do in between? Go back to *primi piatti* (see chapter 4) and stay away from it for a good three minutes, or he'll start rubbing it against your thigh and you'll end up high and dry while your sheets will be soaked.

Marathons

This is when you're pulling out all the stops. You're ready, willing and able to go all the way, maybe even several times. Perhaps the kids are at camp, a blizzard just blew through, or you've carefully cleared your calendar for the next day. You've got lots of time, a preferred partner, and a cache of condoms. Your oral and manual techniques will be the prelude, but the headline act may include a whole series of positions you may never have tried.

CLIMATE CONTROL

In seventh-century China, Master Tung-hsuan painstakingly described thirty basic positions of "clouds and rain," all referring to different styles of intercourse. While you have probably tried a few, we don't know anyone who could come up with thirty. Why, you may ask, would someone want to know about thirty positions for intercourse? Because each one offers different sensations based on the angle and point of entry, and Master Tung-hsuan was thoughtful enough to write them down. While we won't offer thirty positions here, we will tell you about a few angles you may enjoy trying out that will really wow Mr. Stiffy.

Picture your guy on top of you. Some boring guys practice sex the same way they would hammer a nail into the wall—the same motion over and over, only harder and faster toward the end. Some guys swirl around as if they're trying to revive the lambada. He may go in at 45 degrees, then shift into thrusting mode at 90 degrees. Don't make the mistake of continually repositioning yourself so he has a straight shot. Don't always thrust your hips up and down. Mr. Stiffy likes a good workout, where he can stand, bend and move in all sorts of ways. So keep these angles in mind when you contemplate new positions and strokes. This is another chance to show off your newly acquired expertise. Your guy will like the variety, and Mr. Stiffy will love the different sensations.

POSITION TRANSITION

There are countless positions, some of which you, undoubtedly, have tried. Pretty much all of these will work whether Mr. Stiffy is entering through the front door or the back door. You just have to line up the parts a little bit differently, and there are some special tips you'll need to know about backdoor sex. More on this later. The key here is not so much about acrobatics, but refining your skill with a few new twists. Using your imagination, and your buckwheat pillow, will change the angle of entry and give him a workout he won't forget.

In the gay world, we think too much is made of locking partners into being a "top" or a "bottom." Even our friend Phil jokingly said, "I'm a bottom. Let the top do the work: Get it in, get it over with, I want to go shopping." In your old life, you may have had exactly the same sentiments. Scan the personal ads of any gay magazine, and you'll see how tops wear their status like a merit badge, thinking they're in control. Any person, gay or straight, who always envisions him/herself as "giving it," or "getting it," rather than being a partner, is using sex in a way that's weird to us. We think who's on top and who's on the bottom makes absolutely no difference at all.

Everyone knows the missionary position. Try this with

him standing, while you scoot your parts down to the edge of the bed. He can hold your feet in each of his hands and move them higher or lower, separately or together, to change the angle of friction. You can place your ankles around his neck, your feet on his chest with your knees bent, or keep one leg bent with a foot on the bed and the other straight up, resting on his neck. Don't forget to practice your Kegel exercises so that you can give him a tight squeeze inside as well as outside.

A really good in and out stroke that most women overlook is similar to the Princeton Belly Rub (see chapter 10). He's on top in a push-ups position and inside you, both his and your legs are stretched out straight, and his hands should either be on your shoulders or grasping the top of the mattress. Using his tiptoes for leverage, with both of you perfectly flat, he quickly glides his entire body back and forth without raising his pelvis. This rapid rubbing action produces fast results, so you might want to save this for the grand finale.

The Flying Wallenda Position

Another interesting man-on-top technique was inspired by a porno flick that Danny saw. The bottom guy lifted his legs up over his head, the other guy stood above him, and entered the bottom while facing away from him. This seemed pretty tough for straight couples, but we came up with a great alternative, and we named it the Flying Wallenda position. You're on your back, and the guy is in a push-ups position over you, except that his head and arms are between your feet. Bend your legs all the way back so that your opening is facing up, while you hold on to his feet. He enters you from above, and thrusts in and out. If you bench press his feet, it will not only change his angle of entry, but will give you a nice upper body workout, too. The extra bonus here is that your love button will get a nice workout from the weight of his body, and Mr. Stiffy goes in at an almost backward angle for a completely different feeling. Of course, this only works if your partner can measure up.

Hovering Butterflies

If you're feeling particularly gymnastic, try Master Tung-hsuan's Hovering Butterflies position. The guy is on his back with his knees bent up to his chest. You're on top, facing him while sitting on the back of his thighs, with your knees supported by the bed. If you're in this position, the angle changes by him wrapping his legs around your waist. While you have to do most of the work because he's pinned down like a butterfly specimen, he can help you move up and down on his manshaft by placing his hands under your buttocks. This will make his coral stem yearn for your yin essence, and your jade chamber will be pretty happy, too.

T for Two

The T position has you on your back with your legs in the air, with the guy lying on his side perpendicular to your booty. He can hold up your legs and enter from below. In this position, Mr. Stiffy will be coming at you on a sideward slant for yet another new sensation. Gay guys love this because the top guy gets to lean on his forearm and show off his buffed biceps.

X Marks the Spot

Another favorite sideways position, when you both want to lie comfortably on the bed, is the X. All your legs are intertwined; his leg is on the bottom, then yours goes on top of that, then his other leg goes on top of yours. Your top leg can be up in the air or resting on his top leg. You won't be within kissing distance, but the trick with this position is that both partners can vary the pressure by squeezing their legs. This is good if his swelling mushroom is on the small side and has trouble staying in your golden cleft.

Prized Thighs

When a gay guy sits on Mr. Stiffy, he usually does so in a squatting position, and moves straight up and down, giving his thighs a good workout at the same time. But Maggie says that most straight women don't do this; they usually kneel over the guy. Regardless of the position you choose, your partner can put a hand under each of your thighs to help lift you up and down. This will give him more control so, even though he's underneath, he can still pull almost all the way out to get that popping sensation on the ridge of his penis. If he wants to keep his legs straight, place both his hands firmly on your hips. Instead of bouncing all over the place, have him "rub" you forward and back on his shaft. This requires much less energy on your part, and you won't feel like a Pop-Tart. When you're ready for climax, go back to the up-and-down, because that's what really gets him off.

Please Remain Seated While Aircraft Is in Motion

Your sexual arts need not be practiced only in the bed-chamber. If the guy sits on a comfortable chair or sofa, try your thigh-squat position facing either toward or away from him. Both of you will like this because it's so comfortable. Just don't let him get his hands on the remote control, or he may end up watching the football game instead of paying attention to you.

Our friend Don, a chef, once dumped a girlfriend because she refused to have sex any place other than a bed. Maybe it was because of his profession, but for whatever reason, he was obsessed with doing it on the dining room table. When she said no, he tossed her out like last week's lunch special. What is this about kitchens and dining rooms, anyway? We know two guys who had a hot hookup—really hot—because apparently they did it on the stove. If your guy wants red-hot sex, that's fine with us, but stay away from the burners or you might end up as Stove Top stuffing.

One final note: Beware of rough surfaces. As you bounce around on the floor, the sofa, the chair or whatever, keep in mind that even the softest Oriental carpet can leave bad brush burns on elbows and knees.

"A BACK DOOR GUEST IS ALWAYS BEST"

That line is on a plaque outside the back door of a friend's parents' house. For some reason, we always get a little chuckle out of it, considering that the friend's mom is about as uptight as they come. According to our straight friend Don, backdoor sex feels different because of the angle and tightness of the channel. To a guy on the receiving end, the penis stimulates his prostate gland, which can lead to an orgasm. This is not the case with a woman's anatomy. Nonetheless, some women love the sensation, some hate it, and some are indifferent. Several people, gay and straight, have described the feeling of backdoor sex in three simple words: "pain, then pleasure." It's definitely uncomfortable at first, but once your muscles relax and you start moving, it feels great—and this comes from both straight women and gay men.

Massaging the bottom will definitely help prepare you for backdoor sex by relaxing your muscles and stimulating the general area. If the guy wants it, then he should know this, and should be prepared to give you one fabulous body massage before going any further. The most important thing to remember if you're going to try this is that, no matter what, you must add lubrication, because the parts don't get wet by themselves. While he's applying a condom and lubricant to himself, you can put a little K-Y jelly on your fingertips and gently apply it to the outer area, then put a dab or two inside. The guy should know how to do this for you, but you may want to do it yourself to make sure you're properly primed for backdoor action. The next key thing, and this is where a lot of straight guys seem to blow it, is that he must enter you very slowly, stop for a few seconds, and then continue. And, for whatever reason, practice does make it easier each time.

Master Tung-hsuan went on to describe such exotic positions as the Winding Dragon, Bamboos by the Altar, and Phoenix Holding Its Chicken. We think these names are cute, but by adding a few new twists and angles to what you already know, you will become a most honored guest. One of our favorite position stories involves a friend we'll call Margie, who had been lucky enough to have a string of steamy sexual encounters. Leaving the boudoir of her beau, Margie raced out ten minutes late to her weekly yoga class, and came in just as the instructor was telling the class to assume the dog position. Feeling extra perky, and glad that she could figure it out, Margie got down on her hands and knees, pertly protruding her rump. It was then that the instructor calmly corrected her: "I said the dog position, Margie. Not the doggie position."

LOVE TAPS

Love taps are pretty common in gay sex. Just a quick, not-too-hard whack right in the center of the buttock seems to do the trick. The top man will often do this to the bottom during intercourse, and it feels good because the bottom is so sensitized during backdoor sex already. But it will also feel great to the guy on top because you're ringing all his bells at once. You may try delivering a few light taps to your guy during intercourse to see how he likes it. This might be compared to nipple action; he'll either like it or not. But it's a pretty safe bet that no one's ever done it to him before, so why not give it a try?

HOW TO TALK DIRTY, IF YOU MUST

During a sojourn in France, Danny had a wonderful affair with a hot French guy. Between Danny's limited French and the guy's complete lack of English, there wasn't a whole lot to the relationship other than sex, but it was fabulous. The feisty Frenchman had a way with words in bed, and would murmur various French phrases in his deep, sexy voice. Danny loved it, having no idea that the guy was actually saying all sorts of filthy things. In this case, at least, talking dirty was something he enjoyed without even knowing it. Maggie, on the other hand, strongly recommends knowing a little of the local lingo. When a hot Spaniard she was fooling around with moaned, "*Adentro, adentro*," her long-ago Latin training convinced her that "dentro" had something to do with teeth, and she started giving him gentle love bites. Each time he urgently whispered "*adentro, adentro*," she would bite a little harder, convinced that he was loving this. Only later, after consulting her Speedy Spanish translator, did she realize he meant "inside."

Let us continue by saying that neither of us is a big fan of talking during sex, but so many guys seem to get off on it that we felt we needed to offer a few tips. The key thing to remember, and gay guys certainly are aware of this, is that what you actually say doesn't matter at all. Women may long to hear something romantic, but guys are only thinking about their Heavenly Dragon Pillars. It's all about delivery: What turns the guy on is the sultriness in your voice, the low, almost hushed murmurs, the subtle compliments to his manhood and prowess. Talking dirty is one case where you will definitely be performing, so if your guy is into it, just go deep into your method acting and really let go. Deliver your lines in the absolute lowest, sexiest voice you can. If you're feeling really goofy about this, here are some suggested topics that fall into two basic categories. The first deals with him: how hard he is, how big he is, how hot his body is, how he makes you feel so sexy, etc. The second set deals with you: you want him to go faster, to go harder, you love his sweaty body on yours . . . you get the picture. Just don't go overboard, or he may figure you've been getting it on the side at the local truck stop.

So now you've rung all the bells, your yin and yang essences have been released, and your golden cleft and his jade stalk are in happy harmony. Proper gay etiquette says that you should offer him a warm, moist towel before he rolls over and drifts happily to sleep. Not only will he remember your gracious hospitality, but it will keep your Polo sheets from getting crusty.

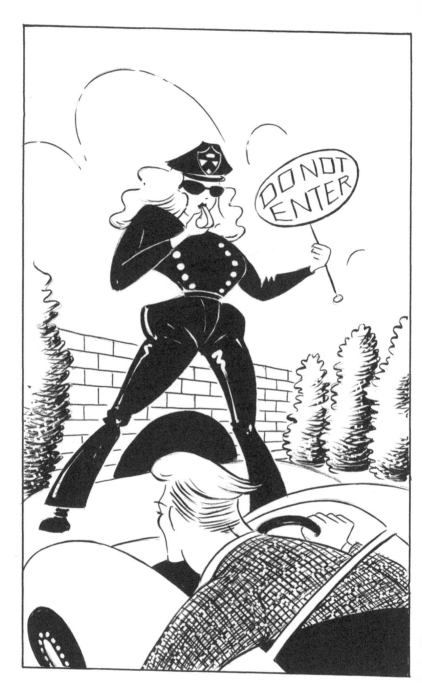

10

"Do Not Enter" Alternatives

Many straight folks seem to think that all gay men do is have intercourse. Not true! Gay guys are masters of the "do not enter" alternative. We can't figure out why so many straight people think that there's no sex without penetration. We know straight men and women who have slept with someone and done everything except intercourse but still don't consider that sex. We think this fallacy might have evolved from traditional notions which dictated that brides be virgins. In other words, the back way was okay, but access to the front door required a ring.

Before the sexual revolution of the sixties, most folks knew that their sexual encounters would probably not end in intercourse. Before a date, guys premeditated their strategy with the precision of a field marshal and plotted every move to get from first base to a home run. They knew which girls would put out and which girls would put them through the ringer before they might score.

Girls knew how to play the game, too. To maintain their reputations, it was their duty to say no as long as they could and still keep the guy interested, notwithstanding his wails of desire and complaints about the dreaded blue balls. Girls also knew that good girls got married, nice girls were popular, and going all the way meant that you were branded the school nymphomaniac, destined for heartache, ridicule and social ruin. If you don't believe us, check out Doris Day in *That Touch of Mink,* or Natalie Wood in *Splendor in the Grass.* Or listen to Meat Loaf's "Paradise by the Dashboard Light." The birth control pill changed all that, and such military maneuvers were as out as white-gloved tea parties. We refer you here to *Beyond the Valley of the Dolls*.

Well, guess what? Times have changed, and the nineties look a lot like the fifties again. Women are gobbling up advice that their mothers rebelled against. The old "good girl" has been replaced by the "rules girl," whose basic credo is "no, no, no" until the ring is on her finger. Whether you're a rules girl, or a party girl, or haven't thought about what type of girl you are in a long time, doesn't matter. There are other, real reasons why "do not enter" has become so popular again. What's more, these activities can be loads of fun, alleviate sexual monotony, and add spice to a humdrum routine. Gay men have elevated them to an art form, so get ready to perfect your pièce de résistance.

SOAP OPERAS

Talk about keeping it clean! Splashing around in the tub can be just as much fun now as it was when you were a kid. Only now there are two of you. Getting into a warm bath together has several advantages: You get relaxed, you get excited, you get off and you get clean. Maggie always thought that erections were impossible in warm water, but after Danny told her about an adventure in a hot tub under the Santa Fe stars, she changed her mind.

The recipe is pretty simple. Find a couple of inflatable neck pillows, run a bath, and add an invigorating herbal scent instead of something flowery. Get inside, relax for a while, and let your fingers do the walking. Add bath gel or mild soap, and let your hands do the rest. Pull yourself closer so your legs go over his thighs, soap up Mr. Stiffy, and go to town.

You can vary the standard bathtub hand job by nestling

behind him. Sit upright while he reclines against your chest. Start with a back, shoulder or head massage while you kiss and lick his neck. Reach around him, or slide your hands under his arms, so that you can nab his nipples. Again, work your soapy hands lower and watch his grower become a show-er. Obviously, this technique works well on you with the positions reversed.

Extolling the virtues of cleanliness, Danny has always been more of a shower person. It's pretty easy to figure out that you can do just about anything standing up that you can do lying down. You can give a guy a pretty vigorous hand workout standing face to face, reaching from behind him, or with you on your knees. Whenever you're engaging in shower action, keep your back to the water so that your face isn't constantly bombarded by shower spray. And don't forget the rubber bath mat. You want him to swoon in ecstasy, but you don't him want to slip and crack his head open. Moreover, your knees will be a lot happier with a little cushioning.

Speaking of being down on your knees, you might want to try some oral action while you're both in the morning shower. Start with hugs, kisses and soaping him up all over. Drop that little inflatable pillow on the floor of the tub, kneel on it, and don't forget to come up for air every once in a while. The water will feel great on both of your heads and, when you're done, you might suggest that he try working with that pulsating shower massager on you.

Maggie fondly remembers a morning-after tryst in the shower with a strapping Norwegian grad student. He had her bend at the waist, arms outstretched, with her hands against the wall for support. Keeping her legs pressed tightly together, he slid his soaped-up shaft back and forth between her thighs. Then he turned her around and continued face-to-face. Swearing that cleanliness and godliness went hand in hand, she rated him "A+" for being such an advanced student.

PRINCETON BELLY RUB

And while we're on the subject of school, let's talk about a drier technique which, in Danny's circle at least, is called the Princeton Belly Rub. When Danny was a student at Columbia, the Princeton boys used to come up to the big city for weekends of fun and frolicking. So many of them were fond of the same technique that it eventually became known as the Princeton Belly Rub. Danny fondly remembers one history student from Princeton who was so good at it that he's earned a treasured place in Danny's personal history.

The basic position is face-to-face, lying down. The guy on top is in a push-ups position, with elbows bent or on the bed. Penises go side by side, and then the top guy rocks back and forth using his toes for leverage. It feels great, and the fellow on the bottom can glide, too, till he finds a spot that's good for him. The beauty of the belly rub for two guys is that they can ejaculate at almost the same time, wash up and head out for a cocktail. For you, it will work best if your legs are open and his legs are straight out, between yours. Then, he can press Mr. Stiffy against your love button. You might try massaging his buttocks or nipples while he's doing this. After climax, just use your nearby hand towel to dry off your belly. This is such a vigorous workout that it's a good idea to make sure you're a satisfied customer first.

BACK SLIDERS

While some women, and more than a few frat boy types, think men will enjoy rubbing their penis between a woman's breasts, we find this unwieldy and virtually impossible for the bosom-ly challenged. A better way of simulating intercourse is called a back slider. This is where you lie facedown on your stomach, while he places some lubricant on your bottom (as opposed to *in* it), between the cheeks. The guy lies on top, or straddles on his knees, and glides his shaft between those golden globes. Like the Princeton Belly Rub, it feels great and is totally safe. Just remember that this is a short step away from backdoor sex, and that if you decide to do that, you'll need more lubricant and a condom.

THE PEARL NECKLACE

Another alternative, which we hear is very popular with both straight and gay couples in the Hamptons, is called the pearl necklace. Danny listened with great fascination as a gal pal in East Hampton told him about an adventure in which the guy gave her a pearl necklace right in the middle of fooling around. "Boy," he thought admiringly, "that's amazing." It was only after he asked her the size of the pearls, and whether they were freshwater or cultured, that he found out what she meant.

This safe and simple alternative has the woman lying on her back with the guy straddling her waist. You can tweak his nipples, stroke his inner thighs, play with his testicles, or play with yourself for that matter. In the meantime, he has his way with himself, masturbating until he reaches orgasm—you can help out by squirting a little lube in his hand—and directing the semen away from your face and onto your neck and upper chest. Hence the name pearl necklace, which can mean any style, from a simple choker to a luxurious opera-length strand, depending on your partner.

This technique is extremely exciting for men because they know how to handle themselves exactly the way they like, and because they never cease to love watching themselves come. It's minimal work for you with maximum return. In theory, the woman doesn't have to do a thing except suggest the whole procedure. He can have a party all by himself, and you can close your eyes and think about the sale at Saks. But you know our feelings on that: no tennis bracelets for sitting around with a bored look on your face. For better results, you should be actively involved, urging him on, with interest and enthusiasm. For variety, you can work in some of your own hand techniques, directing his ejaculation toward the neck, thereby fashioning your own strand of pearls.

M&Ms

M&Ms is the nickname gay guys use for mutual masturbation. It's completely safe; you both get what you want and you can use any preferred lubricant as long as you don't move on to intercourse. Unlike many straight guys, gay men have no problem tossing off in front of their partners. They know that when Mr. Stiffy needs attention, he'll take it from just about any place he can get it, including his old, cherished friend, Mr. Hand. So why do so many straight guys have a problem with handling themselves in front of a woman? Some of the reasons that popped up in yet another of our informal polls included a fear that you'd think he was gay, that you'd think he was a geek if he knew how to toss off too well, that they're obsessed with going "all the way" and won't feel complete unless they do, and that they're just plain lazy and want you to do all the work. (That last response had a slightly bitter note to it; we suggest you try not to think along those lines with your partner.)

One more reason came out when a friend told us about an experience she remembered from college. Seems like one of her girlfriends ended up in bed with a guy and fell asleep. When she awoke, she was horrified to find him tossing off and about to shoot a shot on her. We think she probably shouldn't have been so shocked. After all, boys will be boys, especially in college, and he was probably ready with a story about the dreaded blue balls. But she was out the door before either his explanation or his ejaculation, and the girl told just about everybody she knew. The poor guy became known for his tossing off all around campus, and everybody made fun of him. Maybe it was just college high jinks, but it does appear that straight folks are not quite as comfortable as gay guys when it comes to self-stimulation. This is probably changing, but you still may encounter a little of the old-school shyness.

Sometimes your partner may not have the right touch for you, so you have to take your things into your own hands for a while. The obvious thing is for him to handle himself, too. So how do you, as a straight woman, let your guy know that it's okay for him to toss off? You could try working on yourself, and hope he does the same. You might also let him know that you like to watch him. This is also a way for you to hone your own manual skills by keeping a close eye on exactly how he handles himself. However it happens, just remember that everybody likes M&Ms, and not just the green ones.

COMBO PLATTERS

Just like when you're at the shoe salon and can't decide between the Prada pumps, the Ferragamo flats, or the Blahnik boots, the answer is to go for all three, because you'll always find an occasion to use them. Following the fashion rule of mix and match, you'll want to combine some of your "do not enter" techniques for maximum enjoyment. After some kissing and massage action, get him into position for a little Princeton Belly Rub. If he likes this, he may get close to climax, so be careful not to let him pass the point of no return. Go back to some hugging and nipple action to cool him down for a couple of minutes. Next, have him lie on his back, then it's your option to do manual labor, oral action or both. You can work on yourself a bit during this, too, and he should figure out that it's his turn to do the same to you.

When you both feel really hot and bothered, and you think it's time to let it rip, then move into position for some

M&Ms. Lie on your back, and have him straddle above you on his knees. You may want to work a little of your hand magic on him for a bit to keep things moving. If you haven't yet, put some lube or lotion on your hand or tummy to keep things going smoothly. Try working in some massage techniques (see chapter 4). When you decide you're ready, just start handling yourself. Keep your eyes on him so that he knows you're enjoying watching him, and he should overcome any shyness about tossing off.

WAIT HERE

So your next question is "What do I do while I'm waiting for him?" Even though you may be thinking about how your nails look, it's probably not a good idea to whip out your Revlon and start polishing. Ideally, if you're doing M&Ms, you should both be able to have orgasms at around the same time. In rare instances, however, your guy may take a lot longer than you. If you find yourself in this situation, you'll want to help him along as much as possible. While he's tossing off, whip out all your tips and work on his nipples, inner thighs, buttocks and testicles. He should get a charge out of that. Holding his testicles with one hand and pressing around the base of his shaft in the L formation should also bring him closer to orgasm. If he needs a little more lube, squirt some onto his penis or into his working hand. Maggie swears that you'll encounter this about as often as you'd see Ed McMahon walking up your driveway with a $10 million check. Danny says to see his notes on Pig Dick (chapter 12).

The important thing to remember is that you don't want to seem uninterested in his orgasm, and the truth is, you probably *are* interested in it. He'll like your hands massaging and touching him, so he doesn't feel like he's flying solo. He'll also like it if you gaze admiringly at Mr. Stiffy and give him a warm, affectionate sigh of happiness for a job well done. That way, he'll know you're happy and that it's okay for him to let loose, too. So hold on, relax and enjoy the view.

CALL ME

All this brings us to another set of "do not enter" alternatives where the participants can be across town, or across the globe, depending on your budget. Phone sex can offer a hot and heady experience when both partners go about it with gusto. Unlike those naughty late-night ads on the adult station offering men and women waiting to talk to you, we're talking about phone sex between two partners who are equally involved. You may think, "Why bother?"—but it's something you might try. If you want to get an idea of what it's like, or what to say, try calling one of the gay or straight 900 numbers. Just be prepared with something to tell your husband when he questions the phone bill.

Our friend Margie had several romantic encounters with a guy we'll call Richard, whom we all met in our friendly neighborhood bar. He was handsome, smart, funny and, more important, one of the sexiest guys she had ever met. We had to agree. This guy was such a seductive talker that it took her a while to figure out that he probably had a wife and kids somewhere in the suburbs.

When Margie moved away, Richard would occasionally call for a friendly chat, but the conversation invariably turned to sex. At first, she was reluctant to even answer when he asked her to describe what she was wearing, her underwear, or lack of it, and if she was getting hot while talking to him. She thought it was stupid, but she also found it more than a little intriguing. Richard would describe what she wore and what she did when they met. He would tell her how hard he was getting while he talked to her. He flattered, he teased, he moaned, and he sweet-talked her into putting her hand inside her own panties. While she was no stranger to self-stimulation, Margie had never done anything like this before. But Richard was a master. She remembered the delectable feel of his body on top of her, his large and velvety penis, and his mouth and hands caressing her body. To make a long story short, he was able to talk them both to orgasms over the phone. Whew!

The best phone sex is between two people who have already experienced at least some degree of sex together. Just imagine how hot you could get your husband if he called you one night while working late at the office. Don't use words he's never heard, or refer to things you've never done. If you usually call his penis something cute, he won't buy it when you start calling it a "hot rod to heaven." As with all our recommendations, you need to be an active participant in this scenario, too. Remember, he can't see your face, so he needs to hear it in your voice. You'll also want to make sure that he's as into it as you are, or your conversation might end up being the entertainment at the next Rotary Club meeting.

CYBERSEX

On-line sex chats seem to fascinate many guys of a certain age and with the right equipment. We used to think this kind of thing was just for wonks, but one night, at an upscale, gay party, some pretty sophisticated guys were glued to the computer monitor as digitized nude photos of Brad Pitt appeared on the screen. The guys began to type out a raunchy dialogue with other cybersouls. Most admitted that, every once in a while, they liked to enter the chat rooms on sex.

Cybersex involves communicating with men you've never met. Some guys are content to let their loves live on-line. Our friend Christopher, however, hooks up with guys from the Internet all the time. He agrees to meet them on a certain corner, checks them out on the fly and, if they're not to his liking, keeps on walking. Cybersex may lead to a date, an affair, or even marriage. Just be prepared that your on-line loverboy may turn out be a troll, and not the "SWM, handsome, athletic, professional" guy you expected.

Stiffany & Co.

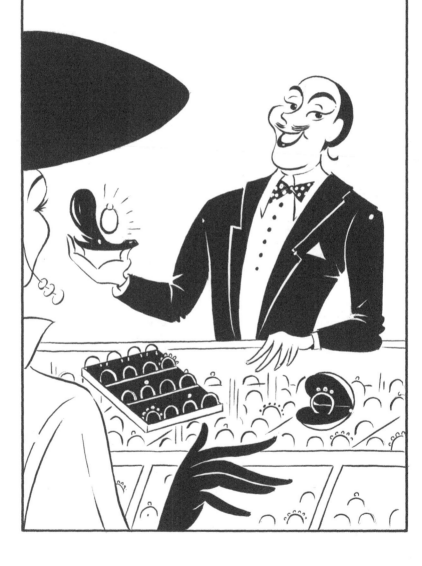

II

Go for the Gold Ring!

Once upon a time, there were two perfectly respectable career women who thought they might like to check out the pleasures of vibrators. It's not that they weren't getting it at home, it's just that they knew that modern conveniences such as food processors made life a whole lot easier, and they both bonded big time with their cell phones. They were ready to try out some new mechanical devices and to spice things up a bit.

For them, manual operation was perfectly fine, they just wanted to see what they might be missing. After all, this was the age of technology, but clicking on to http://youngstud.cum just wasn't their thing, and besides, they felt as though they would be sneaking around in cyberspace behind their husbands' backs. Furthermore, they both had a sneaking suspicion that their spouses might enjoy some new adventures in toyland.

As they lived in a section of the city where one couldn't walk a single block without running into an acquaintance, they let their fingers do the walking through the Yellow Pages, jumped into the car and headed out to the uncharted anonymity of a suburban shopping area, to a place called Pleasure Treasures, for their exhilarating shopping spree.

Feeling very naughty, they walked past the titty mugs, the rolling papers and bongs, the penis pasta, and the NO MUFF TOO TOUGH T-shirts. They briskly bypassed the leather-and-chain section and headed straight for the vibrators. Somewhat overwhelmed by the assortment, they nervously purchased two cheap plastic penis-shaped, battery-operated things, and raced back out to the car.

They eagerly opened their prized purchases and giddily

inserted the batteries to test out their new toys. Checking out the various speeds, they pored over the instructions and poked and prodded each other, nearly knocking their coffees out of the car cup holders. Oblivious to passersby and giggling like two schoolgirls caught passing notes in class, they were having big fun until a loud, determined knock on the window scared the living daylights out of them. They both screamed, tossing up their toys in fear. One vibrator rolled safely out of sight onto the floor, while the other one did a half-gainer right into the coffee, pirouetted just enough to splatter the front seat and our friends, and bit the dust. What a mess, and all for naught; it turned out the man at the window only wanted their parking space.

In fact, the model our two friends purchased may be fine for solo acts, or for performing in front of an audience, but it's definitely not the apparatus of choice for duos. Very few men—gay or straight—are going to be turned on by a molded plastic facsimile of the real thing. Some might wonder whether it's a replacement for them or, worse yet, they'll start comparing it to themselves—inch by inch.

GOOD VIBRATIONS

Instead of the cheapie versions like our friends purchased, we suggest other models that are safer and more powerful, and can be manipulated with greater ease. While the plug-in varieties will require you to stay in the proximity of an electrical outlet, you can always get an extension cord if your activities take you away from the bedroom. What's more, they have variable speeds, which allow different folks different strokes, and are a quick fix if you're all alone on a Saturday night, too. The Panasonic Panabrator and the Hitachi Magic Wand both have knobs at the end of a longish handle. Our straight friend Brett, with years of experience under his belt, preferred the latter. Another model curves around for easy access to your partner, but we can't say we know anyone who's ever used this. If you're feeling squeamish about shopping for toys, most of these models are usually available in many chain stores such as Wal-Mart, CVS and Rite-Aid.

Vibrators can be soothing or stimulating, depending on where you put them. We've already mentioned the benefits of massage in chapter 4. If he seems like the type who likes to be in control, hand him the baton and let him conduct a foreplay symphony on you. He'll be turned on by your moans and groans of ecstasy. You can reciprocate by putting the knob close to his taint during your manual or oral activities; just remember to keep the speed low or else he may buzz right off the bed. During intercourse, the best way for both of you to enjoy one is to position the vibrator on your pubis while the guy is inside you. That way, you both get a buzz at the same time. If you're on your stomach during intercourse, try putting the vibrator beneath you for the same effect. The weight of your bodies will keep it in place. If you're face to face, it's easier for the person on the bottom to hold the vibrator between you. One imaginative friend of ours has a beeper with him at all times for his real estate business. He found that by setting the beeper to silent vibration, he could have a party in his pants all by himself. He also claims that the beeper was the perfect size to slip between him and his girlfriend.

A friend of ours gave us one of those "discreet" catalogs with all kinds of sex toys we'd never even imagined. Our eyes wide with wonder, we stayed up late into the night poring over this catalog of erotic inventions. With everything from Delay Spray to something called the Clitterrific, we were both fascinated and amused. They even had dildo replicas of famous porn star penises. We figure that if you want to strap on one of these, you'll know where to find it. While you're at it, maybe you should seriously consider your sexual orientation. And if he wants you to use one of these on him, our advice is to say "so long" right now. It's only a matter of time until he goes out searching for the real thing.

RING AROUND THE ROSY

Most women and straight guys know very little about the next toy worthy of mention—the cock ring. When one of Maggie's girlfriends worked in an upscale jewelry store in Massachusetts, these were available for purchase, and were sometimes engraved to give as gifts. The last time we checked, however, Tiffany & Company didn't have any out in their display cases. So if you want one, you'll probably have to go your local sex store.

The purpose of these rings is to keep Mr. Stiffy stiff for a longer period of time. Some guys swear by them, but agree the ring is used mostly for special occasions. If you haven't been dating someone for a while, or if you plan to use this on the delivery boy, be forewarned. He may be shocked, begin to sweat, and remember that he has to go somewhere at just that very minute. Worse yet, he may feel intimidated because he has no idea of what to do with it. This toy is better for couples who have been together for a while, and who feel pretty secure about trying new things. If this sounds like your situation, you won't have any trouble introducing new toys. Hand him a small box tied with a satin ribbon. This is a subtle, ladylike way of making the suggestion without ever having to utter a word. His response when he opens the box will tell you what to do next.

You might imagine that this is like playing ring toss over the pole. In fact, Danny used to think that they went over the shaft only, and was surprised to learn otherwise. Despite being informed, and roundly ridiculed that he was quite wrong, he still maintains that this can be just as satisfying, and was pleased to discover that good old Master Tung-hsuan was fond of that usage, too. There are three types of cock rings—leather, rubber and steel—but they basically function in the same way. The guy has to put both his penis and his testicles through the ring. It goes without saying that this is much easier to do when he's soft; it probably couldn't even be done when he's hard. In the same way that most women prefer putting in a diaphragm in private because of all the contortions that are necessary to get it in place, the application of the cock ring is generally done beforehand and alone. But if he's into it, and once it's on, he'll feel very proud of himself, and may start strutting around like a rooster.

Some gay men like to wear a cock ring all day long. The idea is that it's mildly stimulating and is also supposed to make a man's box look bigger and more alluring. One friend of ours decided to wear one while shopping in the city one day. Maybe he thought that he was Jumbo the elephant, or maybe he didn't realize how cold it was outside, but when a cold wind blew up his pants, the darn thing wriggled right off and fell down his trouser leg. Hitting the pavement with a distinctive and embarrassing clink, the ring rolled into the street and was run over by a succession of cars, trucks and buses. Needless to say, Jumbo the elephant turned into Charlie the chicken, and our abashed friend took off faster than a bat out of hell.

Steel cock rings do come in sizes, which is another reason to use them with someone you know well. Guys don't want to find an assorted variety of rings clanging around in your nightstand drawer. You can tell by experience whether he's small, medium or large, so choose accordingly. Most men would prefer that the sizes be large, huge, and humongous. An important thing to remember is that it shouldn't be too tight, otherwise you can do some serious damage. The leather varieties come with adjustable snaps, ties and even Velcro; but these can get pretty skanky and be a real turn-off, especially if he thinks you've used this with lots of guys before him. Another word of caution here. If he likes these so much that he goes out and gets himself a leather band with weights attached, he's primed to look for "rough trade" of the variety that's probably not of your gender.

BOTTOMS UP!

This brings us to a category of toys that are inserted up one's behind. You either like them or you don't. We're sure thousands of viewers remember one episode of *The Newlywed Game* on television. The host, in his inimitably cheerful and patronizing way, asked the contestants, "Where was the strangest place you ever made whoopee?" Two wives gave predictable answers, but the third said, "That'd be up the butt, Bob."

If you're not sure whether or not your partner would be into this, test the proverbial waters by gently inserting a lubricated finger before trying anything else. If he mumbles "um-m" rather than "ugh," he likes it, and it may be time to go shopping at the sex store again. Butt plugs, as they're known in the gay world, come in all sorts of varieties. The most agreeable ones are relatively narrow, flexible, have a rounded top, are covered with latex, and have some mechanism for easy removal. We've heard that there are battery-operated varieties that have been affectionately called tush ticklers, but we have the same reservations about these as we do about battery-powered vibrators. Batteries can corrode, explode, and conk out at the most inopportune moments.

Maggie was once staying at the home of a boyfriend who had yet to firmly commit to his sexual preference. He was sleeping with her, but she sensed he was probably gay. In the middle of a late-night bathroom run, she discovered there was no more toilet paper left on the roll. Sleepy-eyed, she foraged in the cabinet beneath the bathroom sink looking for more paper, and was quite surprised to find a greased-up travel toothbrush holder. Maggie immediately tiptoed downstairs and called Danny for advice at 2 A.M. We sort of guessed what it was used for, but were certainly surprised to find it lubed up and ready to go. Danny told her to put it back and never mention it again. We affectionately remember this as one of the incidents that cemented our friendship.

Do not, under any circumstances, poke something up someone's behind that might get lost. Do not, under any circumstances, poke something up there with a pointed end. It goes without saying, do not poke anything up there that you wouldn't want poked up you! And remember, a little lubricant is key here.

CLIP TIPS

While we pretty much covered nipples in chapter 4, there's another little apparatus that might appeal to you and your partner. Nipple clips can be purchased separately or as a pair attached by an eight-to-ten-inch rubber cord. These basically serve the same function as squeezing someone's nipples hard. Some guys like it; some don't. The sensation of lying on your back, with erect nipples squeezed, while your partner goes down on you can be quite delicious as long as pleasure doesn't turn into pain. Those who prefer the clips with a cord usually like to yank them off in one fell swoop. That seems a little scary to us, but as always, it's a matter of preference. You may be a little nervous about making the formal introduction of nipple clips to your partner. You may want to take them out of your bedside drawer, and suggest that he tenderly place them on you one by one. If he looks at you like you're a freak, just murmur in a hot, breathy voice that you have really sensitive nipples. You can put them on yourself if he's not into it. After he sees how much you like it and how harmless they are, he'll probably be much more willing to have you try them on him. It goes without saying that these should be gently removed before you move into any seriously acrobatic acts.

BETTER LIVING THROUGH TELEVISION

It always amazes us that many women overlook videos—one of the easiest and most accessible devices to turn guys on. You can be squeamish about other devices because you don't want to purchase them, or because you're not into toys; but there's absolutely no reason in this day and age to feel the slightest embarrassment about getting videos. Unless you're in the Bible Belt and the only video store is Blockbuster, almost every video rental place has a section or a room for adults only.

Another one of our informal scientific polls showed that women are more turned on by reading sexy stories than by watching people have sex. Men love to watch. If you don't believe us, think about all those porno theaters and twenty-four-hour peep-show booths that stay in business year after year. Someone's got to patronize them. Nowadays, even the most sophomoric bachelor parties steer clear of live entertainment, whether it's a babe in a big cake or a visit to a brothel. The modern-day alternative is for the guys to get loaded and go back to someone's place to watch videos.

The beauty of video is that you can choose from just about a zillion titles featuring every sexual fantasy you can think of. You can also preview them alone and at your leisure, in the privacy of your own home. This is where it's really important to choose the right stuff for you. If you think something's gross, then watching it with him won't do much for either of you. If you're adventurous, go ahead and see what you like. He'll be so amazed that you did this that he'll be happy with whatever you choose.

For those who find this concept somewhat appealing, but don't want to deal with hard-core, we suggest starting with something that qualifies as sex kitsch. This could be renting an old copy of *Flesh Gordon,* where the hero battles the terrifying space penisaurous, or *Deep Throat,* a classic by any measure. These dated videos are tame by today's standards, but they will get your point across. Other old sex videos are a hoot because of the polyester pantsuits, high hairdos and leather passion pits. Porno titles can be funny on their own: How about such classics as *Phallus in Wonderland, Bimbo Bowlers from Boston, Rookie Nookie* or *Sex Trek: The Next Penetration*? If you don't know where to start, just check out the date on the box. Anything made in the sixties or early seventies will probably be a riot. If you're scared to bring them up to the checkout counter, just casually mention to the clerk that you're having a bachelorette party. No one will bat an eyelash.

Let's say you can handle something a bit racier. While

lots of guys are turned on by watching two women making it together, he might think you're trying to send him a message. Ditto on anything else that you may not want to practice. Guys are pretty easy that way; if you show them something, they'll think you want to do it, too. Choose what's right for you. He'll figure it out.

Okay, now you want to know when to introduce the video, right? We already told you that your VCR and monitor should be within prime viewing distance from the bed, and that a remote control is key. Prepare the videos in ascending order of sexiness. If it's a guy you've known for a bit, just call him up, promise him beer or whatever, and tell him you want him to come over to watch some videos with you. If he asks what you've got, rattle off the list of titles. Be prepared for a moment of hesitation on the phone. Women don't usually do this sort of thing. He may not believe you're telling the truth, but tell him he'll have to come over to find out for sure. He'll be there before you can microwave the popcorn.

Suppose he's a full-fledged boyfriend or husband. Get to a point in the evening where you're both relaxed. You can have the videos all stacked up with one already in the VCR. Tell him you've prepared a surprise for the evening's entertainment and ask him to join you on the bed. If you really want to make sure he gets the point and is having a good time, begin stroking Mr. Stiffy; he'll be out to say hello before the opening credits are finished, and you won't have to worry about another thing.

If the guy is someone you want to seduce after a date, your best bet is to have a naughty little video all queued up and ready to go when you get home. Just invite him in for a drink and casually turn on the VCR, or better yet, hand him the remote. Things will fast-forward in no time, and you'll scoop up one more gold ring while riding his carousel.

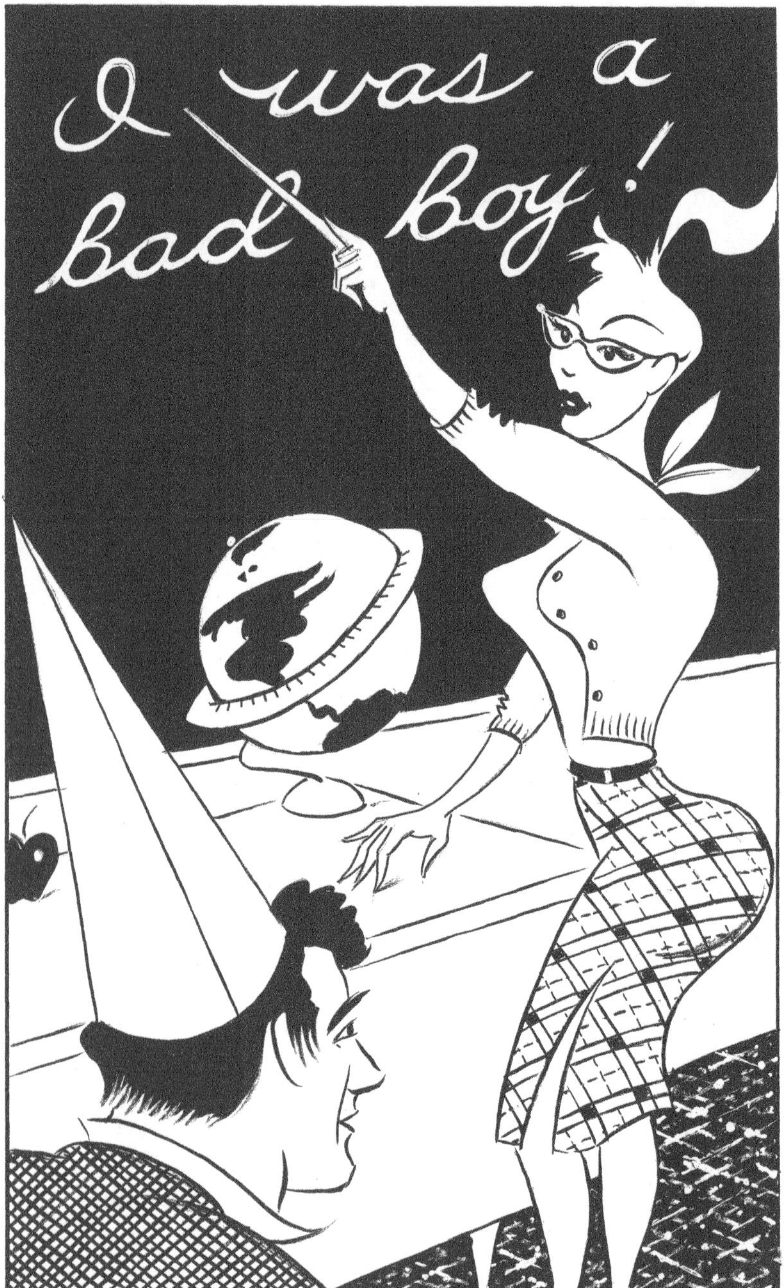
I was a bad boy!

Granted, men are probably somewhat more adventurous when it comes to trying new sex things. Maybe it's because they don't want to seem wimpy, because they watch more videos, or because men just experiment more with their own bodies. Have you ever asked a guy if he's tried to give himself a blow job? We don't know and we don't care. But the fact is that from time to time, even the most willing and playful partners are confronted with frustrating situations, or with requests to participate in something that they're just not into. No matter what, they don't like it, they don't want it and they're just not going to do it. That's what this chapter is all about.

GRACE UNDER PRESSURE

Recently, Philip, a very proper gay friend of ours, said that lots of guys in his crowd were getting into golden showers, and that he had actually tried it. For those uninitiated into the lingo, that means tinkling on your partner. We could no more imagine him doing this than visualize him walking down the street buck naked with a calla lily stuck up his rump. But our inquiring minds did want to know, so we asked him to tell us how he dealt with this request.

It seems as though, in the early throes of passion, Philip's fashion-model partner asked him to pee on him. Our friend said that the guy was incredibly hot, and if it made him happy, it really turned Philip on to please someone else with something so simple. "How could you do that without cracking up?" we asked. While Danny couldn't stop laughing, Maggie asked if they at least got into the tub first.

But we had to grant Philip one thing. Even though we thought this maneuver mixed up form and function, it certainly didn't hurt anyone. Moreover, our friend adhered to the cardinal rule: maintaining grace under pressure.

Being able to keep your wits about you, say no, and still be sexually alluring is one of the hardest things to do. Perhaps that's why some gay men are pretty up-front about identifying themselves in personal ads as "tops" or "bottoms." We generally don't like the idea of categorizing oneself into some kind of posture from which you can never break free, but we do believe in setting your own limits. On the other hand, a lover's request should be considered—at least for a split second. Flexibility is key whether you want to try something new, think about it for a while or bolt for the door. Equally important is what you say when the pressure gets to the point where you want to draw the line.

First, it's important to consider the relationship. There are lovers who are keepers and others who make one very happy that answering machines exist. If your uptight banker husband thinks it would be really great to smear Nutella all over your private parts, we say, why not? Besides having to do an extra load of laundry, there's nothing in this request that's intrinsically harmful, although we suggest that he might get tested for low blood sugar if it keeps up. Ditto for the musician boyfriend who wants to shave your pubic hair into the insignia of the artist formerly known as Prince. You might want to keep an eye on other things that could indicate that he's gone off the deep end. The distinct line between kooky-kinky and a bona fide nutcase should be relatively easy to determine, especially if you've been with a guy for some time.

In a split second, it's up to you to determine what is or is not acceptable to you. We've already mentioned Danny's incident with the vampire from Lancaster. Quiet and repeated murmurs of "no, please stop" did nothing to dissuade this toothsome terror, so Danny was forced to give him a butt in the head. On the other hand, our friend Laurie, a fashion merchandiser, was once handed a spatula by a guy she had dated several times. Initially she had no idea what to do with it. But after he plopped himself facedown on the bed, she quickly understood that he wanted to be spanked for being a very naughty boy. This didn't turn her on in the least, but what he wanted was harmless, and she had a great story to tell everyone on the sales floor the next day.

MAYBE, MAYBE NOT

If a long-term partner suggests something you've never done, but you think you can handle, we think he should be humored and given points for creativity. He's probably just trying to spice things up a bit. Such things include dressing up in slut clothes, sex in the elevator, crotchless panties, shaving, talking dirty, playful tying up, blindfolds, spanking, vibrators, ticklers, edibles, rubber gloves and the like. These may seem odd to you, but all in all they are fairly banal and basically benign.

Ditto on role-playing his fantasies. Laurie is not the only friend who told us her partner wanted a spanking. And the number of stories from gay and straight friends who said their men wanted to tie them up with ties or scarves is too numerous to get into. Fantasy is fine as long as it doesn't become the staple of your sex life. If he continues to insist on lassoing you with a rope and playing ride 'em cowboy, or that you are the fishy and he's got to catch you with his big ol' fishing pole, we recommend you reconsider the relationship.

In most of these situations, the crucial thing is to keep yourself from laughing. Just do what our friend Anthony did: Pretend that you are Princess Grace at a diplomatic dinner where you've just been served fried ants. Keep your composure, indicate your tolerance for foreign customs, and try a taste. Just don't make the mistake of saying, "Wow, this is fabulous. I'm going to get myself a ton of these to snack on every night." Who knows, his little request may be something you can learn to love. Once you've determined that this play is definitely not going to be held over, it's a lot easier to smile sweetly and just say, "No, I don't feel like it." In relatively harmless situations, whether you deliver this line straightforwardly or in a coquettish drawl is purely a matter of personal style. The alternative is to suggest a different activity that may be equally fun. Few men of any persuasion would turn down an offer of a good blow job, for example, especially one from you after reading this book.

READ MY LIPS

If your long-term partner suggests something really odd, such as dripping hot wax on you, sex with the family dog or anything that involves kitchen cutlery, you have a different situation on your hands. "I don't feel like it" is definitely not enough. "You must be kidding" is inappropriate because he probably isn't kidding at all. "That's not my thing" or "I don't want to" are phrases that tell him you're not going along for the ride. Your facial expression and style of delivery are important. Start politely, but progress to a sterner "no" if you have to. Your best bet is to stop something before it starts. If he continues to come at you with a meat cleaver, that's your cue to leave.

Sometimes even long-term partners can conjure up stuff that goes against your grain. If you don't want to be hand-cuffed, have sex with his best friend, have beads put up your bottom, or hook up with another woman while he watches, just say no. If he pouts, says you're too conservative, or tries to force you to do something you don't want to, tell him, "Lay off."

DANCE WITH A STRANGER

Casual liaisons are another story. Sometimes the situation is humorous and sometimes it's not. When our friend Anthony was a young man, new to the Philadelphia gay scene, he found himself at the palatial Main Line home of a well-known, blue-blooded gentleman. They had begun making out, undressed, and instead of heading for the bedroom, the guy marched him into the butler's pantry. Handing Anthony several cans of peaches, he said, "Throw these at me." Anthony didn't have a clue whether he was supposed to open the cans first or not. Figuring that the guy preferred sweet syrup to cold cans, Anthony opened the peaches and artfully aimed them so that the guy was decked out with a pair of peach epaulettes and a tasty tam-o'-shanter. Mr. Blue Blood was so taken with Anthony's savvy solution that he took him to Savannah for a weekend, where they achieved peach perfection.

Use your own good judgment about getting yourself involved with anything or anyone you're unsure of. Paul, another friend of ours, met a guy on the Internet, and they agreed to meet for a drink at what, unbeknownst to Paul, turned out to be an S and M bar. Even though he felt out of place, he was somewhat intrigued by the floor show, especially since, on that night, they were hosting what we can only describe as an S and M Tupperware party. When his date started sampling the merchandise, Paul decided this was one on-line application he needed to exit.

EXIT STAGE LEFT

This brings us to another point. If you're at his place, you can leave. Gay men know to always have cab fare handy in case things don't turn out as planned. Our friend John was in bed with a guy he really liked when all of a sudden there was a loud thump outside the patio door. An odd enough sound, considering that they were in a third-floor apartment, but even odder when John realized the noise was the guy's ex-boyfriend landing on the deck after scaling an outside wall. The spurned ex started pounding on the door and shouting all sorts of mean, unprintable things at John. Armed with cab fare and a quick stride, John was out the door in less than a minute.

Similarly, Maggie was once fixed up on a date with a prominent architect who invited her to his country house for the weekend. Wisely, she made a point of meeting him there in her own car. Things were going really well until he put his hands around her neck and started choking her. When she pried his hands loose and flipped him off of her, he told her she was weird because his former wife loved it. As she put on her clothes, Maggie told him that it wasn't her idea of a good time, and got out of there—fast.

If a guy's at your place, you may have a problem on your hands. Perhaps a bit overimpressed by appearances, a friend of ours invited this Harvard grad back to her place and they started fooling around. Curiously, the same hands around the neck thing happened, but this guy wouldn't leave. He got so angry that he threw an ashtray and shattered a full-length mirror. Our friend kept her wits about her, scooped up his clothes, tossed them out the door, and locked herself in the bedroom to call 911. Lucky for him, he was gone before the cops arrived.

Gay men have an advantage in that their physical prowess is more on a par with their partner's. But who wants to be in a situation where you have to use force? The best advice we can offer is to make your feelings known *before* you get into compromising positions. Maintain your cool and refuse politely but emphatically. Do not crack a smile or he might think "no" means "I can be convinced." If that doesn't work, butt him in the head, show him the door or use your handy glass of ice water to put a damper on his dingle.

COPING WITH FRUSTRATION

Speed Shooting

Premature ejaculation may trouble some women, but gay men don't give this much thought. Why? Because while gay guys want to be memorable in bed, the ultimate object is getting off. So why should they care if he comes too soon or not? But since these tips are designed to make him feel really great in bed, and feeling potent is part of it, we suggest simply getting round one over with and going on to a lengthier, more satisfying round two.

Drunk Dick

Ah, the scourge of partying! This is a tricky situation because there's a point where nothing you can do will charm the snake. In this instance, close your eyes and take a nap. Hung over or not, Mr. Stiffy will probably say hello in the morning, or he might surprise you with an appearance in the middle of the night.

(continued)

Drug Dick

We've pleaded with doctor friends to offer tips on how to counteract the sorry, saggy side effects of prescription drugs such as Prozac and Paxil. Not one doctor could offer a clue. These drugs don't prevent erections, but they can prevent ejaculations. While he may not be able to finish the job, he'll enjoy the sensations you offer with your new hand and mouth skills. Be gentle, be tender, be reassuring, be sexy. Tell him he still really does it for you. But by all means, let him know that you would welcome a little oral and manual motion on you while his parts are in the repair shop. He'll probably feel good that he's able to please you, even if he can't get himself into gear.

That brings us to another category of drugs: illegal substances. We're not talking about hooking up while you're high, or stuff that makes you feel all warm and cuddly. We're talking about substances that lead you to believe you can leap a tall building in a single bound. Why is this a problem? Because a guy can stay hard forever on this stuff. What's worse is they think this is great. This situation is remarkably similar to another situation we've encountered, only this one is substance-free:

(continued)

Pig Dick

There are few things more boring, whether you're a straight woman or a gay man, than waiting for your beau to have an orgasm after you've had yours. While, naturally, we want him to have the most memorable sexual experience of his life, we have run into one or two fellows who may be just a bit of a pig about orgasms. They make you do every move imaginable, and they still won't let it rip. If this sounds like something you've encountered, give it your best shot, but don't be disappointed if your hot techniques are to no avail. Just make it clear by your actions that your hand, or mouth, or whatever is getting a little tired, and that it's time for him to do his thing. If he's already working on himself, don't take over, or he'll never let up. If he absolutely refuses to have an orgasm, then you may want to turn on the TV or light a cigarette to let him know that you consider this performance over.

Schizo Dick

This seesaw scenario has our dear friend Mr. Stiffy up, down, and everywhere in between. Our friend Margie once brought home this

(continued)

young, studly looking guy who worked at an Italian restaurant. He got it up and put a condom on. Everything was fine for a while, but then it went down and he took the condom off. She was very nice about the whole thing—the first time. She was less nice the second and third times. Several hours and a six-pack of condoms later, she decided it was too much effort to even throw this loser out. She went to sleep and made him buy her an expensive brunch the next morning. When the means outweigh the end, cut your losses.

Dead Dick

Sometimes, you might be faced with a flaccid phallus. If it's a first-time encounter, things may just need to mellow out a bit. Except for Danny, who swears this has never, ever happened to him, every guy deserves a break. You've now got all the skills it takes to perform magic. But there will be times when, even if you follow our tips, nothing will awaken the sleeping giant. If this happens to you again and again, start by taking a fair assessment of yourself. If you know it's not you, it's time to consider your relationship to the person in question. Is he a prize fish, or should you catch and

(continued)

release? Dead dicks for long durations have dire consequences. Rest assured that, with your new sexual stratagems, should you decide to ditch, you'll certainly be prepared for the next guy on your dance card.

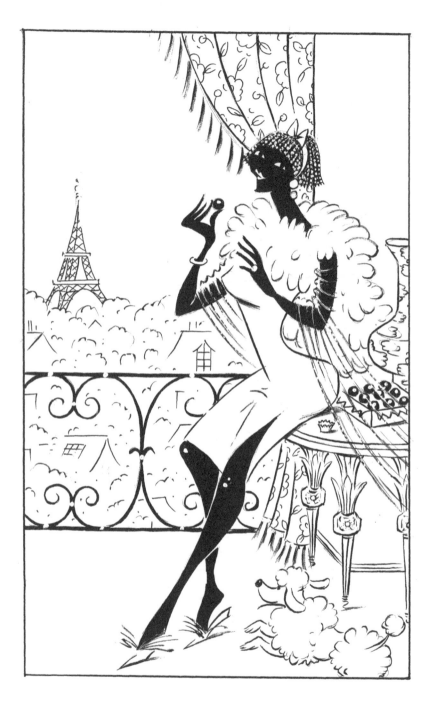

13

How to Get What You Want (Besides a Great Reputation)

Our friend Barbara told us about the time she saw a really hot guy on the New York City subway. They had meaningful eye contact all the way from lower Broadway to the Upper West Side. Her heart was pounding, as the thrill of actually meeting this man intoxicated her. Finally, he stood up to exit at the 96th Street station, and poor Barbara, headed for 110th, watched him leave the train and never laid eyes on him again. What a pity she wasn't privy to the pointers that could help her snag her prey. A few days later, she asked our gay friend Russell what she should have done, and he laid it all out for her. Barbara should have followed the guy off the train—all the way back to his apartment building, if necessary. If they still hadn't spoken, she should have followed him into the building and looked as if she were visiting a friend, maybe even rung some random apartment. Russell figured that if she made it that far, something was bound to happen. While Barbara couldn't imagine being so brazen as to actually pursue this tactic, she had to admire the plan. The maneuver revealed what most gay men already know: If you've got someone in your sights, go for it, and don't stop until you get what you want—or until you decide you don't want it anymore, whichever comes first.

While to some straight folks it may seem that gay guys can't settle down, most will admit to a certain fascination with the gay ability to get what one wants. It's a combination of confidence, luck, timing and the fact that most guys are ready for sex just about all the time. As our dear girlfriend Anna says, "Women need a reason to have sex and men just need a place." True or not, gay men have a whole arsenal of tactics designed to turn chance meetings into tricks—that's gay talk for one-night stands—flings, or even long-term relationships. Now it's your turn to pick up some pointers.

PREMIUM PRIMPING

Even if they're just running out for a drink with friends, gay guys wouldn't dream of heading to a bar without a full primp first. You never know whom you may run into, and you have to be prepared for anything. That's why a facial mask, shave, shower and deep conditioner for the hair are absolute musts. You'll want to do all of this, too, and even though a gay guy might be shaving his face, and other parts, you'll know what areas you need to tend. This could also explain why gay men are notoriously late, although they never miss an appointment at the tanning salon. That's because knowing you look good makes you feel great, and when you feel great you're ready to be fabulous.

Sometimes, we have more fun during primp time than when we actually do go out. First, we'll open a bottle of champagne, or mix up some gimlets, then start with the facials. Gay buddies may watch a Bette Davis movie during this phase, but we often opt for Marilyn Monroe, Lauren Bacall or *I Love Lucy* reruns. Next, we'll head off to the showers for shampoo, scrub, shaving and makeup. Most gay guys never wear makeup, but a little tube of cover stick can come in handy when faced with a monster zit or dark circles from too much dancing the night before. Then it's time for the hair products.

Our friend John has a very elaborate method of doing

his hair. After a shower, he sits with a de-bouffing baseball cap on for exactly fifteen minutes, then he applies a leave-in conditioner with his hands—he wouldn't think of using a comb—and leaves that in for five minutes. Next, he blow-dries his hair with an old seventies brush dryer. Then he adds a few quick curls with his curling iron, affectionately known as Wanda, followed by major hair spray. Of course, any over-the-head clothing has been put on long before the spray to avoid any mussing. One time, John insisted we simulate the lighting in the club we were headed for so he could be sure his hair shine would dazzle the crowd.

OUTERWEAR AND UNDERWEAR

Gay guys spend as much time determining their outfits as someone else might do strategizing the winner of the Kentucky Derby. Starting from the inside out, they pick their underwear with the attitude that someone else may see it, and you should do the same. Squeezing yourself into a super-spandex bodyshaper may be fine if all you have in mind is for people to gaze at you, but not if you're ready for serious action. Danny has his favorite flannel boxers, and Maggie has her cranberry lace duo. You should know what's right for you.

Select clothing carefully, because you can be sexy without looking like an ad in *Hustler*. You want to show off your best features. Danny wears black turtlenecks or blue oxford shirts to show off his blue eyes. Maggie wears a short skirt to show off her legs. While gay men always know exactly what's in style, straight guys don't have a clue. They only know if you look good, so work it.

Even if it's freezing out, gay guys never take an overcoat into a club. If there's no coat check, then they'd have to drag it around with them all night, and who wants to worry about losing a cashmere coat while on the dance floor? Worse, who wants to make a hot prospect wait while you stand in line to get your wrap? If you're driving, leave the coat in your car, or just jump in a taxi and hope that you'll be in someone else's limo on the way home.

One last note on dressing: Another of our informal polls shows that all men—gay and straight—detest large handbags and backpacks, especially in a bar or club. Our friend Charlie remembers a woman he was ready to move on one night. Unfortunately, she kept shifting her gigantic handbag from floor to lap to bar and, according to his description, did an absurd-looking Mexican hat dance around her bag on the dance floor. Stuff your necessities into a pocket—either yours or a guy friend's—or find a small bag you can deal with easily. Save the suitcase for when he flies you to Acapulco for the weekend.

CRUISING AND SCOPING

There's a slight difference between cruising and scoping that is sometimes blurred in conversation. Cruising is what straight people think gay guys do all the time: hunt for other guys to pick up. And that probably is what most of us think when we use the term; there's definitely a sense that the cruiser is looking for action, and soon. Scoping, on the other hand, is a much more subtle and creative endeavor. You can scope just about anyplace and, in fact, you have probably done it lots of times, you just didn't call it that. You can scope out a bar, a dance floor, a rock concert or a Bach concert. The basic act is the same: a quick but inclusive survey of all the potential "menergy" in your sightlines. No meaningful eye contact here, just a short, not obvious, glance in all directions. All gay men learn scoping at an early stage as part of their coming out; soon it will be second nature for you, too.

Street scopes, better known as "gaydar," are like radar on the road. Any gay man can tell you about the scope, stop and turn. You're walking down the street and see another guy; you both check each other out as you walk past each other. Then what? Keep walking, count to three and turn around. If he's interested, he'll do the same. Sometimes, it will happen three or four times and you'll be almost a block apart. It's very exciting at this point. You can decide that your coffee date with your best friend is more important, or you can turn around and start walking toward him. He either waits for you to catch up or starts heading back toward you. Out of politeness, Danny always opens with something like "Didn't I meet you at Stephen's party last month?"—even when he knows darn well that he's never laid eyes on the guy before. Sometimes you'll get a date for later, sometimes you'll never see him again, and sometimes you'll end up calling the coffee shop to let your friend know that you can't make it.

Say you enter a bar. The initial scope is important because it will determine many of your next moves. Before you actually move into the throngs of people, you pause for a brief moment and do your subtle survey. Where are the people who are having the most fun? Where are the geeky losers? Where are the bar trash types? You should be able to answer all these questions in a single sweep. So the next step, unless you have some sort of fatal attraction for geeky losers, is to head right in the direction of the fun part of the room. These are the people you want to be near, and while you can't exactly crash their conversation, it's much better to be near them than near all those high-hairs huddling in the back. The other factor to consider is optimal viewing positions, both in terms of seeing and being seen. You don't want to end up in a dark corner where no one can see you, and where you can't have a good view of the action.

Gay bars are usually designed a lot better than straight bars in terms of scoping. The circular scope, sometimes called a twirl, is Danny's favorite way to check out the lay of the land. The circular scope is simply a walk around the entire bar, and in gay bars, at least, you can almost always do a full circle without running into a dead end. The circular scope can be solo or with a friend. If you go with a friend, don't forget to stop every couple of minutes, toss your head back and laugh out loud. That way, everyone will know how much fun you are, and they'll also figure out that you and your friend aren't an item. If you're in a bar with a male friend of any persuasion, it's superimportant to keep scoping the room so other guys know you're unattached. The scope is particularly useful in bookstores, gyms, art openings and Starbucks.

TARGET PRACTICE

So while you're on a twirl, you see an attractive guy whom you wouldn't mind hooking up with. He looks your way, and now comes the meaningful eye contact phase. Just look right back at him for a good bit—say, five seconds—smile ever so slightly, then look away. The next time you look in his direction, voilà, he's looking back, and you do the same thing all over again. This can go on for quite a while and, admittedly, can go on for absurdly long periods in gay bars. Chances are that since he's a guy and you're a gal, he'll make the first move. You can facilitate this by heading in his direction and ordering a drink nearby. If he's smart, he'll step up and buy your drink. Otherwise, keep him in your sights and continue with the eye contact. Check out what he's drinking. This is also a good time to check out his pants, shoes, and any accessories to make sure he's up to your high standards.

If he's really hot, buy him a drink. This can be done two ways. The first, which can be a lot of fun, is to have the bartender deliver the drink to the guy. Usually the bartender gets all into it and loves doing it, but Danny ended up with a disaster one time when he described the guy's outfit very carefully to the bartender and nodded in the guy's general direction. All of a sudden, some other guy wearing the exact same thing swooped on to the scene and landed the complimentary cocktail. It happened so fast that the poor bartender didn't even know he'd given the drink to the wrong guy. Danny decided it was time for a twirl, and the hapless impostor never did find out where the drink came from.

The other, safer, way to buy a guy a drink is to order it

yourself and hand it to him. At least this way, you can be sure the right guy will get it. He'll probably be so shocked that you did this that he'll be a bit speechless, so you had better be prepared with a good opening line after you say, "Here, I thought you might like this." Just remember that all you did was buy him a drink, and you shouldn't assume that because he accepts he has to sleep with you. If he opens his mouth and sounds like a dirtball, feel free to end the conversation politely and head back to your friends. Remember, never be rude in a bar, because the guy you snub tonight could be your job interviewer tomorrow.

CLOSING THE DEAL

In business terms, the guy you end up meeting will be a "qualified lead," meaning that he's already shown some interest in you, via eye contact or whatever, and that you have a good shot at landing him, if you want to. As in any business, however, closing the deal is tough. We've said before that part of your new sexual persona is the confidence that you *can* have what you want, and once you get it, it'll be the best ever. Danny has had numerous encounters where they end up at his place after a date, then talk until the wee hours of the night. Eventually the other guy says, "It's late, I'd better be going." Danny says, "Fine," then walks him to the door, they chat for a few more minutes, and then the goodnight kiss turns into a marathon make-out session.

This may work well for you, too. If you don't want to let the guy into your place, the decisive moment still comes at your apartment door. The fact is that someone has to make the first move, and it might as well as be you. As we've said, gay guys don't usually have to worry about taking the lead, and neither should you. Knowing what you want is important, too. If you make it to the door and decide you don't want a make-out marathon, then just say "Good night," and let him go. The point is that you have to take some risks, and if it doesn't work out, you have to be ready to move on to the next one without looking back.

Seductive gestures and conversation are skills worth honing, but don't overdo it. Danny has a strategically timed stare, head toss and chuckle. Other guys swear that casually running a finger back and forth over the lower lip works like a charm, and girlfriends have reported some success by using the same gesture with a neckline. Subtle is the key. Keep your ears open for a lead-in. If the guy says, "I don't want a relationship, I'm just into fooling around right now," you can say, "Me, too." This may sound idiotic, but guys throw stuff out to test the waters. Once they think that you tacitly agree, they feel much more comfortable about taking the next step. According to our friend Fred, this technique has landed him two long-term relationships, not to mention more than a few evenings of great sex. When all else fails, remember the cardinal rule— just grab it!

HAVING IT YOUR WAY

Those sitcoms where the wife says, "I've got a big surprise for you when you come home tonight," might sound funny on TV, but that's not the way to get what you want. You'll do better if your suggestion can be acted on at that very moment. Throughout this book, we've told you how to stroke, massage, tickle and titillate. Starting with a soft, sultry voice, a few eyelash flutters and, most important, a couple of touches to his arm, inner wrist, hand or thigh, will undoubtedly get your intentions across. Getting what you want in bed is not all that hard. Women often let the guy take the lead in the beginning, and the guy wants to show off what he can do. Fine, let him. Just remember to "ooh" and "coo" at what you like. He'll get the idea.

Sometimes, a guy might be a pig and not think about what you want. Gay guys have the advantage of being able to do exactly what they want done to them on the other guy. We still recommend this technique as the best one for getting your point across. But sometimes, like when you've been married for a while, or have fallen into a humdrum routine, you have to be a bit more explicit. That's when it's important to know how and when to ask without sounding like a professional.

If you want him to do something he's done in the past, but seems to have forgotten about lately, just murmur, "I really love it when you . . ." or "Thinking about (fill in the blank) really makes me wild." To get him to try a new position, just do it. To get him to try a new technique, you might try saying that you had this incredible sex dream the night before, and describe what you wanted and how you reacted. Don't even give a second thought that he'll think you're a tramp. Men love sex a lot, but he'll love the fact that you want great sex with him even more.

A WINNING WAY WITH WORDS

Some folks love to talk during sex, and others can't stand it. We both fall into the latter category, and could no more utter "Do it to me hard, baby" than drive naked down the L.A. freeway. Gay guys make a big joke about the inane dialogue in porno flicks. But some people, guys especially, get a charge out of talking during sex. If you feel like you have to say something, see chapter 9. Just keep it short so it doesn't sound like a lecture. More difficult is shutting him up if he insists on talking and you want to fantasize about Tom Cruise. The best technique is to plant a kiss on his lips and keep it up till he gets the point. If that doesn't work, try lightly running your fingers over his mouth and whisper, "Sh-h, I love to hear your heavy breathing." If you want to get more graphic, tell him you love to hear his man-grunts, but we would certainly have a hard time doing this with a straight face.

AWARDING REWARDS

Gay guys rarely say anything positive or negative about their partner's performance, because everyone involved knows whether the sex was good, lousy or off the Richter scale. Most guys would prefer saying nothing, rolling over and going to sleep, but some women think they have to give a postgame wrap-up. Again, the key here is keep it simple, like "Wow," or "That was great." Your moans and heavy breathing will let him know what really turned you on, and if you are happy. But if you want to know whether or not to fake it as a way of reinforcing good behavior, the choice is up to you. Just be assured that he can't tell if your contractions are voluntary or involuntary, so do what you please; Mr. Stiffy will be none the wiser. Mr. Stiffy, and your partner, will be so ecstatic with your new sexpertise that you'll be the one who's getting the trophies.

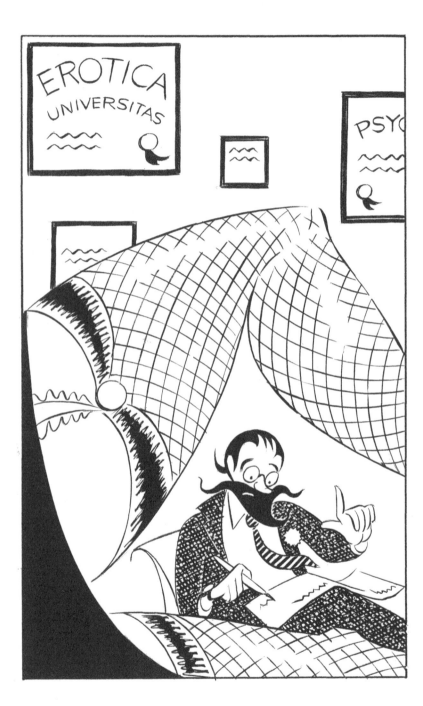

14

Dear Dan

COMMONLY ASKED QUESTIONS AND ANSWERS

Dear Dan: Do "blue balls" really exist, and, if so, what are they?

    Blue in the Bayou
    New Orleans, Louisiana

Dear Blue: I've never had them, but my friend Philip claims that he almost died from them once. He was all prepared to hook up with his boyfriend after a long absence, and then drove several hours to the beach. He was young at the time, and got so excited during the ride that his balls basically froze up and became so supersensitive that he couldn't even touch them. He says that blue balls are the result of delaying ejaculation too many times. Even after the long ride, sex was out of the question. All poor Philip could do was go to sleep and hope for a fresh start in the morning.

Dear Dan: Every time we have sex, I close my eyes. I think it would be a real turn-on to watch my boyfriend masturbate. How do I tell him I want to watch?

    Eyes on the Prize
    Watch Hill, Rhode Island

Dear Eyes: 1. Open your eyes. 2. During your manual labor, guide his hand toward his penis, then start masturbating yourself. He should get the hint.

Dear Dan: This might sound like a weird problem, but my boyfriend's penis is really huge. I can get it inside my

vagina, but there's no way that it fits in my mouth. What do I do?
    Trixie Slim
    Big Sur, California

*Dear Trix: Believe it or not, this is not an uncommon problem.
Do the best you can by moving up and down the sides, and try
to get just the tip in your mouth. Use your hands on his shaft,
and save your mouth magic for his balls and thighs.*

Dear Dan: I've kissed a number of guys with facial pierc-
ings, but what do I do when a guy has rings through his
nipples or nether parts?
    Perplexed About Pierced
    Woods Hole, Massachusetts

*Dear Perplexed: For starters, steer clear if you've got braces
or you might end up entangled in the ER. Pierced nipples will
already be erect, so tweaking them with your tongue or teeth is
exactly what he wants. Pressing on a taint ring during manual
or oral action puts pressure on his prostate—perfect for guys
who prefer these pleasure hoops.*

Dear Dan: I really love sex in the a.m., as it makes me
feel great before I go to work. The trouble is that my
husband really had bad breath in the morning. Is it poor
etiquette to suggest he get up and use some mouthwash?
    Breathless in Boca
    Boca Raton, Florida

*Dear Breathless: Yes. Remember what we said about setting
the stage. Better etiquette would be to have a handy tube of*

Binaca spray under your mattress. Spray some in your mouth, tell him to open up, and spritz some in his mouth, too. Then just grab it! I bet he'll never even mention the breath spray.

Dear Dan: I've got this guy who has been my friend for a long time. We go to parties together. We spend Saturday nights together. We watch videos together, eating popcorn with my head in his lap. It's really frustrating because he never does anything sexual. How do I turn this friend into a lover?

Platonically Peeved in

Potomac (Maryland)

Dear Peeved: Just grab it!

Dear Dan: If I go down on an uncircumcised guy and his penis isn't hard yet, do I pull back the skin so the top shows or do I put my lips around all that skin?

Flustered by Foreskin

Frankfurt, Germany

Dear Flustered: Try putting your lips around it and gently play with the foreskin with your tongue; then push the skin back, hold the base, put it in your mouth and prepare for the great awakening.

Dear Dan: You used to be able to tell by the wet spot, but now that guys use condoms and peel them off after sex, I don't know if they really had an orgasm or not. Is there any way to tell?

Doubtful in Dallas

(Texas)

Dear Doubtful: I was shocked to learn that more men, gay and straight, are faking orgasms these days. It just didn't seem like it would ever be an issue, but then I read an article about a straight guy who fakes it the first time around so his girlfriend will think he can do it twice. Nonetheless, if your guy grunts and groans, and then jumps up to flush it down the toilet, you'll never know for sure. If he falls asleep immediately, he either had an orgasm or was too tired to begin with.

Dear Dan: I think the guy I've started going out with is gay. He's a responsive lover, and works his butt off in bed. But I just have this nagging feeling. How can I know for sure?

Wondering in West
Hollywood (California)

Dear Wondering: It sounds as though you have nothing to complain about, but we understand that sometimes it's just nice to know. Maybe the guy doesn't know, doesn't want to know or simply hasn't come to terms with things yet. There are a few things, however, that offer pretty good clues. Check out his CD collection. Does he have recordings of Broadway musicals, or groups like Nine Inch Nails? When he has you over to his place, does he serve canapés and Lillet, or pop open a couple of brewskies? Does he have more hair and beauty products in his bathroom than you? You can't argue with the evidence.

Dear Dan: I can have multiple orgasms. Sometimes my partner wiggles around after orgasm to make it happen a second time. How long does a guy take before he can do it again?

Impatient Lady
Grand Rapids, Michigan

Dear Impatient: Notwithstanding those little blue pills, assuming your guy actually does have an orgasm, figure it will take him about zero to five minutes if he's in his teens, five to ten if he's in his twenties, ten to twenty until he hits about forty. After that, you'd better count on taking a shower, washing and drying your hair, and doing your nails in between—three coats of polish!

Dear Dan: I love having oral sex with my boyfriend, but he never goes down on me. Is there anything I can do to make this more enticing to him?

Delta Queen
Beaver Dam, Wisconsin

Dear Delta: Stop going down on him.

Dear Dan: I really like this new guy I've been seeing, but his penis turns me off. What should I do?

Grossed Out in Grosse
Pointe (Michigan)

Dear Grossed: That depends on how bad it is compared to how much you want him. If the good outweighs the bad, just close your eyes and think of Brad Pitt.

Dear Dan: My boyfriend is mesmerized by those booty-

licious babes in music videos. How can I make him
dance to my music?
>Rhythmless
>Shaker Heights, Ohio

*Dear Rhythmless: Pretend it's Halloween. Put on some boots, a
black bra, and some black shorts or undies and saunter in front
of the TV like one of the Pussycat Dolls singing "Buttons" or
"Don't Cha." Walkin' and talkin' trash gets 'em every time.*

Dear Dan: I am lucky to have a really passionate partner,
but sometimes he's so overenthusiastic that I feel like I'm
in some gymnastics competition. I want him to relax so I
can close my eyes and fantasize. How do I tell him to be
smooth instead of being a cheerlead?
>Pooped in Piscataway
>(New Jersey)

*Dear Pooped: Gay men know to take the cue from their partner.
We generally get the idea that if our partner uses a light touch,
then he likes a light touch. I should think this would work for you,
too. Try putting him flat on his back while you gently massage
him and work some manual-oral action on him. Unless he's totally
dense, he should figure out that you might like the same tempo.*

Dear Dan: Is there any real use for pubic hair? My husband thinks it would be sexy if I shaved or got a Brazil-
ian, but I think I need the hair for a buffer.
>Sick of Lady Schick
>Sharpsville, Indiana

Dear Sick: Pubic hair functions as more than a buffer. The close concentration of texture actually keeps a warm scent in one place and, according to an anthropologist friend, was nature's original design for attracting the opposite sex. Whether your partner likes you hairy, hairless, or with heart-shaped pubes is purely a matter of aesthetics.

Dear Dan: My boyfriend has this thing for putting food you-know-where. I'm no prude, but most of the stuff ends up on the sheets, and I feel like I'm sleeping in a garbage pail. What's the word on food?
    Fed Up in Fruita
    (Colorado)

Dear Fed Up: Gross! Gay men don't do this, and why should you? Tell him if he's hungry to stop at Burger King on the way over.

Dear Dan: Some married friends have asked if I would join them in a three-way. I'm game but what's the etiquette?
    Three Wishes
    Triadelphia, West Virginia

Dear Three: Any gay guy will tell you that the pleasures of the three-way are best enjoyed by the "plus one." But sex with a couple can be tricky. You not only want to tantalize them with your technique and dazzle them with your diligence, but you also want to play fair without losing friends in the process. Keeping your eyes closed prevents playing favorites because you won't know whose lips are locked on your love button and, better yet, you won't care. Chances are that you'll be treated like visiting royalty. But decline a sleepover, as you never know what drama may erupt in the morning.

Dear Dan: Lately I seem to be at parties where the girls end up giving BJs to the guys. It seems one-sided but I don't want to be left out. How can I be memorable without seeming like an overly experienced slut?
New Old School
Collegeville, Pennsylvania

Dear New Old: There's nothing slutty about taking pride in your work and doing things well. Distinguish yourself from the pack. Hold your head high, take a deep breath, and pause for a second before beginning. The trick is to convey self-respect along with respect for his most precious part. Then put one hand in the "L" formation, the other around the base, and go to town.

Dear Dan: What are some good lines for an Internet sex chat room, and how can I tell if the guy on the other end is old enough to vote yet?
On-line in Onancock
(Virginia)

Dear On-line: Chat lines, by their very nature, are designed for fantasy, so go wild. Just make sure you don't accidentally send one of your sexy sign-ons to the office e-mail. As for your second question, if he talks a lot about Avril Lavigne, you can bet he's barely got a driver's license.

Dear Dan: I went out with this guy and saw his body for the first time at the beach. He was really hot, but his back and shoulders were covered with more hair than a monkey. How can I politely suggest he get rid of the fur coat?

Jungle Judy
Tarzana, California

Dear Judy: Get him a gift certificate to your waxing salon. Throw in a massage while you're at it, so he doesn't feel too put out.

Dear Dan: Help! What if I'm at a hotel and don't have my usual nightstand accessories?

Trysting in Trieste (Italy)

Dear Tryster: Ask him to run down the hall for ice. In the meantime, get your glass of water ready, tuck your condoms under a magazine, and move the mini-battle of hand lotion from the bathroom to the boudoir.

Dear Dan: Is there any way to keep sex fresh after several years of marriage with kids?

Hitched and Hot
Long View, Kentucky

Dear Hitched: The tips in this book will undoubtedly put a tiger in his tank. We've always felt that your best shot at great sex is usually with someone you've loved for a long time. So reserve some grown-up time, impassion your partner, test these tips, and have a great time!